TO RAE - my patient wife who never entertained yoga
and the like in her own life, but who was to watch my
full-time involvement in 'alternative medicine'. She
could not precisely put her finger on why it was
abhorrent to her, but when at length fear came, God
spoke to her. 'Trust Me', He said. She heard Him
clearly and was at peace again.

*But the natural man receiveth not the things of the Spirit
of God: for they are foolishness unto him: neither can he
know them, because they are spiritually discerned.* (1
Corinthians 2:14).

More Understanding Alternative Medicine

Holistic Health in the New Age

Roy Livesey

New Wine Press

New Wine Press
PO Box 17, Chichester, PO20 6RY

Copyright © Third Edition, 1988 Bury House Christian Books
First Published by Bury House Christian Books in 1983 under the title
Beware Alternative Medicine; Second Edition, 1985 (Marshall, Morgan,
and Scott/New Wine Press)

All quotations are from The Authorised Version Bible

Printed and bound in Great Britain by
Courier International Ltd, Tiptree, Essex

ISBN   0 947852 08 5

Contents

therapy, art therapy, music therapy,
holistic cosmetics, Bates eyesight
training, sound therapies, hydrotherapy,
aromatherapy, macrobiotics, zone
therapy, orgonomy (Reichian therapy),
bioenergetics, do-in, Feldenkrais
technique, rolfing, mora therapy,
orthobionomy

hypnotherapy, hypnosis, self-hypnosis
tapes, meditation, transcendental
meditation (TM), contemplative prayer,
autosuggestion, Couéism, visualisation
therapy, mind control, quieting reflex,
passivity, centering, guided imagery,
chromotherapy, biofeedback, the
placebo, psychotherapy, psychoanalysis, autogenics, dream therapy, aversion
therapy, metamorphic technique, primal
therapy, inner healing, Rogerian
therapy, encounter therapy, gestalt,
psychodrama, transactional analysis, co-
counselling, clinical theology, transpersonal psychology, psychosynthesis,
group dynamics, group psychotherapy,
interpersonal relationship, positive
thinking, positive confession, positive
mental attitude, human potential
movement

spiritualist healing, psychic healing,
faith healing, hand healers, absent
healing, magnetic healing, healing with
magnets, psychic surgery, witchdoctors,
shamans, charming of warts, copper
bracelets, crystal therapy, pattern

Foreword

In January 1986 The Journal of the Christian Medical Fellowship published a review I wrote of the 2nd Edition of 'Understanding Alternative Medicine'. The review was far from uncritical and I recorded reservations, but I urged the worldwide readership of Christian doctors: "This book is important and I recommend you read it".

Since then Roy Livesey and I have been in correspondence and we have both moved our positions. God does reveal Himself to those who seek Him, sometimes only one step at a time, and we have both progressed. Roy has recognised the deception in some of his previous extreme charismatic thinking and has a much more balanced view in this area. I have moved further. Re-reading the 2nd Edition and reading the 3rd Edition more than two years later, I find myself recognising more and more how the Devil's lies have influenced our culture, our churches, and our medical practices, orthodox as well as alternative. Roy is right - more right than I realised before.

Were I to review the expanded and improved 3rd Edition (and hopefully writing this foreword makes it unlikely!) I would still make minor criticisms. That is natural. I am a doctor with a scientific, academic concern for truth - Roy is an informed, intelligent, deeply spiritual Christian layman who was given by God the job of being a watchman and sounding the alarm about alternative medicine. We may have reached our now similar conclusions by slightly different routes but I am unashamed to stand with Roy Livesey in declaring that the Devil is active in much of alternative medicine. I know of others besides myself who were helped by the previous Edition of this book, and I pray and believe God will use this Edition to help even more.

This book is important and I recommend you read it.

Andrew Fergusson

(Dr Andrew Fergusson B.Sc, M B, B S, M R C G P is a General Practitioner in a Medical Mission in South East London and an Elder in a Brethren Assembly).

Introduction

Nearly twelve months were spent as a full-time 'searcher' in the forbidden area of occult 'healing'. Prompted by terror and horrifying experiences, I was led by a long-standing clergyman friend to a Christian who had a particular understanding of the crisis point I had come to. He was the first really to get through to me with the consequences of my involvement in the innocent-sounding areas of 'healing' and 'alternative medicine'. That was my first introduction to the man who became my pastor. Looking at all the dangers, I was led to the idea that I must be born again.

I didn't understand what all that really meant. Yet when that happened Jesus Christ became real to me. I had invited Him to become my Saviour and Lord.

Not long after that, God put it on my heart to do two things. I had to give my testimony to my old colleagues in 'alternative medicine'. I was able to tell them my life had been totally changed. A peace and satisfaction had come to me through knowing Jesus. Secondly, I had to expose Satan's counterfeit healing to all.

This then is a *warning* book. I do not pretend to have all the answers nor am I condemning all the alternative therapies mentioned in this book. Rather it is my purpose to encourage Christians to exercise their own caution, enquiry and discernment. The occult is on the increase but the Lord is revealing to His people the truth about various practices. The testimonies on homoeopathy are examples.

Without discernment, Christians can be led into occult 'alternative medicine'. Sadder still, without knowledge of the evil in it, there can be no possibility for us to alert those who are blind and cannot see and to whom things of the spirit appear as foolishness (1 Cor. 2:14).

The book does not pretend to be a work of great scholarship! Prayerfully written, it is none-the-less an urgent book. Taken from my own testimony, and from what Scripture reveals, it is at least a book by one who has travelled the way of 'alternative medicine'.

The thief cometh not, but for to steal, and to kill, and to destroy: I am come that they might have life, and that they might have it more abundantly (John 10:10).

November, 1983

Second (Enlarged) Edition

Christians in Britain receive many warnings about *cults*, drawn from the vast experience in the United States. Since the first edition was written, I have travelled in the United States, listening, and speaking at many Christian meetings on the subject of alternative medicine. I believe the greatest experience of the phenomenon is to be found in the United Kingdom. The explosion in occult medicine has happened here. Unlike in America, under British common law anyone can set up as a therapist, provided only that he doesn't claim to be a medical doctor.

The Second Edition is much bigger than the first: over one hundred therapies are included, some harmless, but the great majority having a harmful spiritual basis. Yet I fear there may be insufficient here to satisfy one of the well-known reviewers of the First Edition: '… isn't it time that a group of Christians with the theological, scientific, professional and medical qualifications plus the gift of spiritual discernment, wrote an authoritative and weighty book on this subject?' Perish the thought!

I trust my Christian readers will find that, with God, things are really not so complicated. I believe they will find much here to help them exercise the discernment that God will give them.

A change has been made in the title for this Second Edition, and the significance of alternative medicine in the New Age is brought into focus. Perhaps inevitably, there will be the tendancy to look for what is written about this or that therapy. However I believe an *understanding* of alternative medicine will be helped by reading steadily through the book. The context in the New Age, and in the expansion of interest in the occult realm, will be more clearly seen. I believe such an approach will be an aid to discernment on any particular treatment. The main purpose of the book is to encourage readers to strengthen their own discernment.

June, 1985

Third (Updated) Edition
Alternative medicine continues to increase in popularity. I view the situation even more seriously than when writing the Second Edition. The hold that alternative medicine is taking increases and the therapies themselves are, I believe, generally *more* deceptive than I had supposed.

However there is no purpose in making changes in what has already been written about this or that therapy. Christians are getting their own discernment *from the Lord*, and this book is to encourage that.

The infiltration into the Christian Church runs deeper. For example whilst more are renouncing homoeopathy as occult I gain the impression that more Christians are beginning with this subtle deception than are leaving it behind and renouncing it.

When the First Edition of this book was written in 1983 I hadn't paid my first visit to America as a Christian. I hadn't recognised what is now so very clear both here and in America, the existence of the New Age movement. I had been a New Ager but I hadn't properly understood the vastness of the New Age, and I didn't call it by that name.

I had been a New Ager long before I became taken up with supernatural healing and holistic health. Yet it was holistic health, alternative medicine, that eventually gripped my attention more than anything previously, and it was this that Satan eventually used to seduce me squarely into the occult realm.

When the Second Edition of this book was published in 1985 I was far from understanding fully the relevance and breadth of the other New Age deceptions in our day. Then *Understanding the New Age - Preparations for Antichrist's one-world government* was published in 1986. This was really a Volume Two when it comes to exposing Satan's work through the New Age movement. *Understanding Deception - New Age teaching in the Church,* published in 1987, dealt with the infiltration of the New Age including Holistic Health and Healing and was truly a Volume Three in the same series.

What I didn't at once realise as I proceeded step by step, volume to volume, was that alternative medicine, notwithstanding it was extraordinarily significant in my own course of deception, was indeed a most logical place to start. Alternative medicine is an occult entry point for greatly increasing numbers. Most are interested in their health. It was ever so as man has focussed on himself and his own body. Whilst the analysis in this book can be viewed quite simply by those who have the Holy Spirit and to whom these things are not foolishness (1 Corinthians 2:14), unredeemed man is faced with a vast range of alternatives which mostly appear to be very different. Satan appears to present a marvellous choice. However Christians can see the same threads running through the vast majority of therapies identified. God will give discernment to those who love the truth and seek it only from Him.

In this up-dated edition we take a more detailed look at

homoeopathy. Such is its grip on many Christians, I hope that the larger chapter will be helpful in striking a chord with more people, bringing home to them both the deception and the folly of what really is perhaps the most facile among therapies.

A broadly similar conclusion on homoeopathy was reached by the working party set up by the British Medical Association (BMA) to look into alternative medicine. Their conclusions on alternative medicine generally, though come to from a different perspective, are substantially in line with those presented in this book. They give a general 'thumbs down' for alternative medicine and I include various findings from their report.

There are included guidelines for a systematic approach for considering particular therapies and an application of this to Transcendental Meditation.

Herbal remedies are looked at at the outset in Chapter One. Herbal remedies are biblical. Whilst most of alternative medicine is well avoided by Christians, what we have in this book is *not* a blanket condemnation and I hope that what I have written about herbal remedies may encourage Christians in an area which increasingly seems to be taken over by New Agers.

Perhaps the most serious area for concern and for our discernment is the infiltration of New Age healing methods and techniques into the Church. 'Signs and Wonders', Psychology, Visualisation, Inner Healing and Positive Confession come into this category, and whilst they are looked at more fully in my book *'Understanding Deception - New Age Teaching in the Church'*, the urgency is now identified here also.

Finally, as Christians, shepherds and sheep alike, I want to emphasise the purpose of this book. It is to encourage the reader in his own discernment. I believe a start is made when we realise, all of us, that we *can* be deceived.

For such are false apostles, deceitful workers, trans-forming themselves into the apostles of Christ. And no marvel; for Satan himself is transformed into an angel of light. (2 Corinthians 11:13-14).

How you read this book is very important

Satan and his work is revealed. He would seek to blind us against the truth of God's Word on occult 'alternative medicines' and false healers - Satan's counterfeits of God's true work of healing.

Jesus Christ paid for our freedom, and victory over Satan, with his life. So pause now, and pray that God will open your eyes to all the truth and that He will give you the help you need in order to act on what you know to be the truth.

Note. Whilst this book clearly identifies areas of so-called healing that are quite certainly occult it is emphasised that the main purpose is to encourage Christians to be discerning. Many names are mentioned in the course of showing the variety, and giving a picture, of the alternatives to what the doctor offers. However, just as orthodox medicine is not always free from the demonic, so 'alternative medicines' are not necessarily powered by the demonic. The mere mention of an 'alternative medicine' in this book is not to be taken as any suggestion that it is occult.

PART ONE
BEWARE! THERE ARE
'HEALERS' ABOUT!

There shall not be found among you any one... that useth divination, or an observer of times, or an enchanter, or a witch, or a charmer, or a consulter with familiar spirits, or a wizard, or a necromancer. For all that do these things are an abomination unto the Lord... (Deuteronomy 18:10-12).

Today's sorcerers, diviners, white witches and spiritists are busy 'healing'. It is only the names that are different. Satan has had a plan since Adam, and his demons are as busy now as they were then.

- **Whether** we look at the 5,000 year old 'secrets' like acupuncture, reflexology and meditation, **or**
- **whether** we look back only 500 years to Paracelsus, **or**
- **whether** we look back 150 years to his follower Hahnemann who gave us homoeopathy, **or**
- **whether** we look at the newest techniques or some of the therapies at new healing centres,

what we find is spiritual power rooted in the occult.

1
Some basic questions answered

Do these occult healing methods work?

They very often do work. If it suits his purpose Satan will 'heal'.

He is unknowingly invited into lives through these 'healing' methods; his price is a devastating one. Our religion, whether in the churches or outside, is for the most part humanist with little idea of the supernatural, whether it be God or Satan. So the question 'does it work?' has the wrong focus. The enormous dangers are missed.

In this secular society few doctors deny the experience of the occasional miracle! It is easy to put it down to God when no scientific reason can be found! Science, and a vague idea of God, are convenient blinds used by Satan. What is really happening to the rest of him as one part of man is being 'healed' by Satan?

In one case a woman with depression was prayed for in a Spiritualist Church. She received temporary relief, but she began to suffer from arthritis. In my own case I was cured of haemorrhoids by a spiritualist 'healer'. This fired my enthusiasm for spiritual power. I soon believed that after death I would return to earth in another body. Thus like so many spiritualists I was led to believe in reincarnation. Satan's wiles had blinded me to the truth of an eternal life spent in heaven or in hell.

One spiritual method is much the same as another, and

a big growth area is acupuncture. This is rooted in Taoism, a Chinese spiritual philosophy for which divination was the basis. Divination is spiritual discovery by forbidden magical methods (Deuteronomy 18:10). Also there are more and more 'healers' who can bring a powerful occult touch to an otherwise acceptable practice. One case involved a dental surgeon who treated what he saw as energy imbalances (like the sort deriving from Taoism and seen in acupressure) whilst the patient sat in the dental chair. When he is invited in, however unknowingly, Satan will leave something that was not bargained for.

'But I'm a Christian, and I'm feeling better for my 'healing', so am I OK?'

The seed for physical, mental, emotional and spiritual problems is sown by Satan when given access through occult healing. For a born again believer the walk with God is restricted or blocked as darkness takes over from light. Frequently you hear: 'I don't seem to be able to pray in the way that I used to'.

For someone not born again of the Spirit of God, involvement can mean missing the real blessing that God has. In every case it is only the relationship with Jesus Christ, and the call that can be made on Him, that can undo the damage caused. Satan seeks to deceive us all.

Where do we find Satan's 'healing' taking place?

Don't even go looking! Any involvement is a sin. Occult means 'hidden', and according to God's word it should not be investigated. *My* big mistake was to become a 'searcher' into occult healing methods.

'Healers' are to be found everywhere. Some of the most caring people are wanting desperately to bring something they think is good to the world. They are being led into occult techniques. Many are becoming spiritual (or psychic) 'healers' who consult the dead. The truth is that they are not consulting the dead at all. The dead go to heaven or to hell, and the Bible allows no possibility of communication. Demons impersonate the dead and they are deceiving them.

This 'healing' is increasingly found in thousands of front rooms, in Spiritualist Churches and even in some churches where the focus is on healing and not on Jesus Christ. It is found too in 'Healing' and 'Help' centres opening up throughout the country.

What about herbal remedies?

In previous editions of this book I wrote that some *herbal concoctions* may well be appropriate subjects for enquiry and research. However, simple *herbs*, used in their own right since Bible times can have a God-given healing quality. Straightforward herbal remedies according to Scripture are legitimate and increasingly overlooked opportunities in health care.

Nevertheless, I received several extraordinary letters asking why I *didn't* approve of herbal remedies, and of course I *do* recommend them. '... *the fruit thereof shall be for meat, and the leaf thereof for medicine.*' (Ezekiel 47:12). Given an opportunity, the evil one will blind some to the truth of God's Word. Herbal remedies are indeed provided by God.

What I wrote previously I repeat in the chapter on 'so-called physical therapies', that further enquiry is worthwhile where herbal mixtures are founded in magic, where formulae are given by divination, or where herbs are collected as charms are recited. What we don't want are herbal remedies with which the evil one has tampered. Satan likes to begin with something good.

'Back to Eden' is a voluminous classic on the health to

be found in 'herb, root and bark', written by Jethro Kloss in 1939. The author reminds us that people have been diverted from the true healing remedies by superfluous advertising and false science. Indeed today, and for a long time now, people have been seeing the effects of drugs and are looking for something better, but is there a danger that the once well known herbal remedies are becoming lost to us? At least have they been lost from our attention? How far has Satan progressed with his attacks on God's herbal remedies?

'Back to Eden' reminds us that herbal healing was the first system of healing that the world knew, and that herbs were mentioned many times in the Bible. Jethro Kloss tells us that as a small child he gathered many of them and was taught their use. The scripture teaches those using herbs that they should learn to know the herbs growing around them, and the need to avoid using herbs that can be poisonous or in quantities that will be harmful. In 2 Kings 4 we read that there was famine in the region around Gilgal, and one of Elisha's company went out to gather herbs. He found a wild vine and gathered some of its gourds. No-one knew what they were but into the stew it went! *'So they poured out for the men to eat. And it came to pass, as they were eating of the pottage, that they cried out, and said, O thou man of God, there is death in the pot. And they could not eat thereof.*

But he said, Then bring me the meal. And he cast it into the pot; and he said, Pour out for the people, that they may eat. And there was no harm in the pot.'' (2 Kings 4:39-41). God provided the answer. Men were learning.

My own grandparents and parents learned these things too, yet today surely valuable knowledge is being fast replaced by remedies that the evil one has corrupted. Men hear less from God and more from the diviners that abound in alternative medicine and who follow ways that are detestable to the Lord (Deuteronomy 18: 10:12). Not falling for today's deceptions my Mother, having worked in a manufacturing pharmaceutical chemists in the 1920s and experiencing the herbal and the chemical side by side, still seeks out the stores that will sell the unadulterated remedies, ones she learned about in her own Gilgal experience. For these are nature's remedies, put there by the Creator and pointed to in His Word.

We can seek them out in a prayerful and discerning way. They are still there today for those who will read and learn.

Yet a word of caution must be added. Not all herbs are good for human consumption and we do well to heed a doctor's warning (from America): "As herbal utilisation increases, medical magazines report more and more syndromes associated with their use affecting the central nervous system, respiratory system, the skin, cardio-vascular system and metabolic system." ★ and according to one American Medical Report there is still "a very limited state of knowledge of herbal chemistry and potential toxicity. The extreme variability in the chemical composition of the plants, their preparation, labeling, and marketing, makes buying a particular herb a highly uncertain and potentially risky enterprise." ★★ "Herbal teas can have more serious effects than the caffeine in regular tea that people are trying to avoid. Herbal teas are blends that may contain more than twenty different leaves, seeds, and flowers, so a wide range of toxic manifestations may occur. 'Panacea Tea,' for example, combines morning glory and catnip, both hallucinogens. Anaphylaxis and death have resulted

★ *Holistic Health - A Medical and Biblical Critique of New Age Deception* by Jane D Gumprecht, M D. (Ransom Press, Moscow, Idaho, U S A - 1986)
★★ Report in *Hospital Physician 18, No 10: The Pernicious Panacea: Herbal Medicine* (U S A)

from drinking teas from chamomile heads or chrysan-
themums.''★

We need to remember too that Health Food stores are
substantially infiltrated with New Age thinking. The
spread of vegetarianism is encouraged by similar
attitudes, attitudes that have prevailed in Hinduism for
centuries and which are surfacing in the New Age in our
day. As Christians we can still be guided by the Word of
God:

> *"Now the Spirit speaketh expressly, that in the latter*
> *times some shall depart from the faith, giving heed to*
> *seducing spirits, and doctrines of devils ... and*
> *commanding to abstain from meats, which God hath*
> *created to be received with thanksgiving of them which*
> *believe and know the truth"* (1 Timothy 4:1-3).

The whole world where the evil one rules "lieth in
wickedness" (1 John 5:19) and Jesus is not Lord in
Satan's earthly kingdom. Readers of the remainder of
this book need be under no illusions. Satan starts with
something good. The vast majority of alternative
medicine serves Satan's purpose. His purpose can be
subtle; they are certainly significant in the New Age.

★ *Holistic Health - A Medical and Biblical Critique of New Age*
Deception by Jane D Gumprecht, M D. (Ransom Press, Moscow,
Idaho, U S A - 1986)

2
The current thinking

'Healing' and 'Help' centres

There is a fast growth of these centres where occult healing methods are included in the range of alternative treatments. These centres may be residential, or not. They can be profit-making or voluntary. They are not of course to be confused with the Medical Centres where the medical profession is to be found, but they are increasingly gaining credibility, support and approval from influential people.

In these stressful times man is full of uncertainty about death; whilst he is alive he is full of uncertainties about his health. Satan knows this. Anxieties remain whether the staff at the Centre are charming and friendly or whether they are not; whether the treatment is free or expensive; and whether patients actually 'feel' better or whether they don't. More important: when the occult is involved, the 'extras' and the 'approval' only serve Satan's purposes. The care, the good diet, and the peace of the place only encourage patients to continue. Whatever the outward appearances, Satan moves into any establishment where an occult technique gives him an opening. Satan is no respecter of persons. Spiritual activity not in line with the revelation of the Bible, and not in Jesus' name, is an open invitation to him.

What do today's leaders have to say?

Slowly a public awareness is dawning even if based mainly upon the horror stories that abound following experiences with the occult. The Bishop of Gloucester wrote in his *Diocesan Gazette* (July, 1983) about false and corrupt perversions:

> 'They are not sanctioned, and in many cases are roundly condemned, by scripture, Christian tradition, and reason alike, and Christians are best advised to steer well clear of them all from horoscopes and ouija boards to seances and so-called healings by means of occult practices or magical devices.'

Then beneath the Bishop's message, and as if to evidence the spiritual warfare being waged in these days, there appeared a private letter lifting up a cancer help centre as a place glorifying to God. At that centre treatments described in Part Two of this book are practised. The *Gazette* reflected both sincerity and confusion. Man's reason and tradition need to be supplanted by God's wisdom if Satan's schemes are to be stopped.

Sincerity in these matters is irrelevant. A sincere person unknowingly on the devil's side, is a dangerous counsellor. Satan is real. He is alive. He is very sincere! He knows God's word inside out. Ignorance of it is no defence. The truth is in God's Word, *not* in man's sincerity, *not* in man's traditions, *not* in man's reasoning and *not* in any of man's ideas about what he thinks is good. Ministers often say 'Focus on God'. That's right as far as it goes, but we can't afford to ignore Satan. Ministers often approve of yoga and of divining (whether for water or for 'healing' purposes). They have been deceived. Yoga and divination are spiritual; indeed yoga is a form of worship. Such things are 'detestable to the Lord'.

Paracelsus was a very famous occultist, animist, alchemist, diviner, astrologer and magician who lived 500 years ago. Like most today he did not look to God. He looked to himself and the natural world for his remedies. He unknowingly joined Satan's side in the spiritual war. He pointed to nature as the source superior to the Bible. The deceptions of Paracelsus gain ground today. The scholarly encyclopaedias enable Christians to identify Paracelsus as a man working with the counterfeits defined in Deuteronomy 18:10-12. However, and in distinction to the message of this book, read what the Prince of Wales, then President of the British Medical Association, told the doctors at their conference in December 1982:

'But what kind of man was Paracelsus? A charlatan or a gifted healer? In my view he was far from being a charlatan. In this, the 150th anniversary of the B.M.A. we could do worse than look again briefly at the principles he so desperately believed in, for they have a message for our time: a time in which science has tended to become estranged from nature - and that is the moment when we should remember Paracelsus. Above all he maintained there were four pillars on which the whole heart of healing rested. The first was philosophy; the second astronomy (or what we might now call psychology); the third alchemy (or bio-chemistry) and the fourth virtue (in other words the professional skill of the doctor)'. He then went on to outline the basic qualifications for a doctor: 'like each plant and metallic remedy the doctor too must have a specific virtue. He must be intimate with nature. He must have the intuition which is necessary to understand the patient, his body, his disease. He must have the ''feel'' and the ''touch'' which make it possible for him to be in sympathetic communication with the patient's spirits. Paracelsus believed that the good doctor's therapeutic success largely depends on his ability to inspire the patient to confidence and to mobilize his will to health. By the way, he also recommended chastity and fasting to heighten diagnostic sensitiveness and to intensify one's hypnotic power!'

In the five years that have ensued since Prince Charles' speech we have seen increasing credibility heaped upon Alternative Medicine. However no Paracelsian philosophy, no royal or clerical approval, no measure of care or concern can counter the great and inevitable dangers in store for those who fall for the wiles of Satan.

The growth of the occult in Britain was helped in 1952 by the repeal of the Witchcraft Act. This made Britain one of the most liberal countries in the Western world. More recently the World Federation of Healers was granted government approval to treat patients in NHS hospitals. The Federation comprises largely professed mediums.

It will remain to be seen whether alternative medicine is to become a political issue in Britain. The costs are low compared to what the NHS can offer from medical science, and many of the unemployed are setting up as therapists. Michael Meacher, MP, then the Labour Party's shadow spokesman for Health and Social Security, seemed to put his weight behind the movement when he opened the Alternative Medicine Exhibition in 1984.

On the international scene, at the United Nations in 1973, the much-respected World Health Organisation (WHO) recommended that the medical profession accept the validity of native cures like those used by witchdoctors. The place of the WHO in the end-time scenario is looked at in Chapter Seventeen.

The truth of what God says borne out by experience

Kurt Koch is a recognised authority on sorcery and demonology. In *Occult Bondage and Deliverance* he writes that anyone who enters Satan's territory, however unknowingly, will immediately be harassed by the powers of darkness. They will feel the effects in different areas of life. He described Harry Edwards as one of the most dangerous healers in the Western world. He writes that he has come across thousands of cases in which contact with the occult was the root cause of the problem. In nine out of ten cases it was clear occult involvement had played some part.

3
Discernment

Jesus wants us to repent of our sins and to seek a relationship with Him. He wants us to be born again and to take the power and authority that are available in His name. Until that happens there can be simply warning in this book. However when we turn to God 'like little children', there can be revelation of what is written here and on what is written in Scripture.

But the natural man receiveth not the things of the Spirit of God: for they are foolishness unto him: neither can he know them, because they are spiritually discerned. (1 Corinthians 2:14).

But the comforter, which is the Holy Ghost, whom the Father will send in my name, he shall teach you all things, and bring all things to your remembrance, whatsoever I have said unto you (John 14:26).

The Scriptures are for today. By the power of the Holy Spirit they can speak to us today.

The spiritual dimension: the problem of the intellect

There is relatively little written about Satan's involvement with 'healing' and that is as true today as when the First Edition of this book appeared. One of the problems is with the intellectual aspects. Also most of those who have looked into Satan's spiritual realm in a deep way are still there in that place. As far as I am aware, all but one of my many friends and acquaintances from the days of 'healing' are still there - in that same spiritual realm. The deceived cannot be witnesses.

When a patient is 'healed' of a complaint and says he is better or that he feels better, even the believer can have difficulty in speaking out against it! That 'Satan himself masquerades as an angel of light' is a truth to which we believers seem easily blinded. On top of that, the intellect has to deal with the mixture of science and nature, of God and Satan, in the proliferation of 'alternative medicines' that are available. How do we explain our lack of joy when Granny or one of our dearest friends tells us of a release from pain, since the acupuncture, since the reflexology or since she went to see 'that nice lady' who laid hands on her? We can only seek God's guidance in each situation.

There is no intellectual explanation in terms that Granny will be likely to understand readily, and there is even some danger in explaining what acupuncture needles are supposed to do. They will be deceptive explanations. The intellect will understand the needles, the energy flows and much else from the acupuncturist's explanations. The intellect will often marry them up with some understanding of science. The true intellectual and spiritual explanation will present difficulty to those whom Satan has involved. The idea of an occult root will present a problem to Granny or to our friend, whatever their natural level of grasping problems might be. In the spiritual dimension we are concerned both with the root in the history of a particular discovery and with any occult involvement of the practitioner himself. Any intellectual exercise can be useful only when directed to finding this out.

The surest answer is given to the spirit that is right with

God. Seeing that the promoters of alternative health methods are fast gaining recognition by medical science it becomes increasingly necessary to check the spiritual status of those who treat us.

Discernment

Discernment is essential in a Christian fellowship. I believe discernment is given when the need is there, when we are open and seeking to receive. I believe we have to begin! Having taken the first step more will be given when we show we are prepared to trust God and receive. As Christians we often act on this witness of the Holy Spirit in our own lives but we then can deny God by passing it off as intuition. Often I hear: 'I would steer clear of acupuncture (or whatever) but I don't know why'. Of course Satan can pervert anything, but most often I believe Christians' intuition is of God! When we acknowledge Him, He will often confirm it; our confidence is built up, and we move on. God gives us more. Confronted by mountains of deceptive information, often we don't dare recognise that it's God's voice (and why shouldn't it be when we are moving in his Spirit?). We stand aside and watch 'alternative medicine' grow.

These are urgent times and it is clear that enormous numbers of people across the world are coming into the spiritual dimension. Many are coming to know Jesus as Lord and Saviour and so experiencing the indwelling of the Holy Spirit.

On the other hand there is a rapid acceleration in the growth of the occult - not only 'alternative medicine' but everything occult.

Children are coming into the spiritual dimension before their parents, through drugs and through rock music and discos. However, the Holy Spirit is giving Christians a new awareness. Rock music is an example.

It has been at last rumbled by discerning Christians! How could Christians have been blinded for so long? Some of the lyrics actually praise Satan. Many a Christian Mum and Dad has neglected to see what their children are into. We are offended by the noise and the behaviour so we keep away. We don't of course see the drugs our children use. We don't hear the lyrics. We don't understand the spiritual significance of the beat, and we wrongly suppose it isn't significant. We don't understand the effects of the strobe lighting and we have perhaps never endured it long enough ourselves to see its effects. The fantasy world effect is increased by the smoke effects but the undiscerning may simply regard it as unpleasant. The truth is that the kids receive the beat and the lyrics even if they themselves aren't aware of them. Satan understands! Ask the witchdoctors in Africa who call up spirits with the same beat!

Many hang on to 'Christian' rock but the Holy Spirit is moving through this whole area. This is still a controversial area among Christians. However, consider what is common to *all* rock music. An occult beat and certain strobe lighting effects cannot be neutralised by Christian lyrics whether they are clearly audible or not.

In the world's view, rock and disco are far removed from the quiet of Transcendental Meditation looked at in detail in Chapter Six. Taking a spiritual view, they have everything in common! The extremes of noise and peace are hardly the relevant factors. In both we 'switch off.'

Satan is into everything! The Bible says he is the ruler of this world (1 John 5:19). Discernment is essential. Jesus won the victory over Satan. However, Satan still has to be taken very seriously by Christians. Power over him is given to those who will receive it, and in order to know the enemy when we see it, God gives His people discernment.

'Focus on Jesus' doesn't mean 'ignore Satan'!

The battle is against Satan (Eph. 6:12). Therefore we must not ignore him. The discernment we need to identify him is not an intellectual exercise. It is given to the heart or to the spirit, and Satan would cloud it at the first opportunity. Yet he is more than an opportunist; Satan is a planner!

An easy way to play into Satan's hands is to continue to talk his language. It serves Satan's purposes to speak of 'seeing Granny' when what someone has seen is a ghostly ectoplasmic manifestation of Granny created by demons. It serves his purpose to talk of energy lines when talking about acupuncture. They don't exist. The ghost of Granny wasn't Granny either! Granny is spending her eternity with the Lord if she knew him. Otherwise she is spending it separated from Him. Either way, Scripture allows no opportunity for her to return. Satan brings about these manifestations according to the access he has gained and the faith in him. How much better to have that faith that comes by hearing, and hearing by the Word of God (Romans 10:17).

It is often heard (and it is said to me): 'you talk too much of Satan'. Often people can't say the word 'Jesus' before they come to know Him. Indeed typically there is surprise at hearing the name of Jesus except when used blasphemously. Satan wants to stop the use of the name because there is power in that name. By the same token, among Christians, Satan doesn't want his own name mentioned. In fact Satan would like the whole spiritual dimension to be unknown. I was forty-four years of age before I knew that dimension existed. I might have talked about it as I had talked about Jesus, but I didn't know that dimension in either realm, and I didn't know Jesus. I was *en route* to hell without even knowing it.

We can speak without fear about Satan. Satan deceives undiscerning Christians with the suggestion that to speak of him is to glorify him. On the contrary it is glorifying to him when we ignore him, or accept his deceptions. Satan is the father of such lies and manifestations. It is the way of the world ruled by Satan to receive the counterfeit faith and to glorify him by acknowledging his lies. The Bible tells us to put on the armour of God. It tells us to receive the true faith that comes from hearing the Word of God.

Certainly occult 'alternative medicines' are not for discussion apart from prayer. The narrative for each therapy in Part Two of the book has been kept to a minimum. Not all the therapies are known to me; the Holy Spirit counselled on what was needed for my walk with the Lord. He always gives the same answers to those who seek.

May God give his body the much needed discernment. May we receive also from him the help needed to act on the truth revealed to us, and may the truth be broadcast throughout the Church.

Before looking at particular techniques and schemes

Satan's schemes extend to all of us. He tailors them to our lifestyle. The most dangerous techniques among the 'alternative medicines' are as dangerous as the ouija board and tarot reading.

It cannot be over-emphasised that there is nothing that is really special about any particular technique where the occult is involved. They all involve faith in something supernatural, Satan and not God. When someone in every street is into acupuncture, it is easier for the unbeliever to turn to acupuncture! Satan can accommodate us (and get an entree) with anything we put our faith in that is not of God.

Jesus said '...*ye shall know the truth, and the truth shall make you free* (John 8:32). The truth is in God's Word.

Occult alternative medicines are summed up in one word — Satan. Satan knows all about science too; he's in on it! The spiritual warfare is hotting up and the only way to fight the battles is with the weapons and armour that God provides (Ephesians 6:10-18). However, the guide to various therapies that I have included in Part Two should be helpful. This was written after some prayerful consideration to determine how far to relate Satan's deceptions and 'so-called deep secrets' (Revelation 2:24). Romans 16:19 also tells us: *'for your obedience is come abroad unto all men. I am glad therefore on your behalf: but yet I would have you wise unto that which is good, and simple concerning evil.'*

Not all 'alternative medicine' is founded in the occult; I believe most of it is. The task of the discerning Christian is to sound the alarm or the 'all clear' as the Lord leads. It may seem unfair to include the medicines and techniques against which there is no evidence. But, for example, who knows which 'herbal concoctions' might be OK? God knows. If we earnestly desire to know, we can listen to Him.

Looking at particular therapies

In following their profession medical doctors are familiar with the ways of eliminating all the possibilities before coming to a difficult diagnosis, and they are used to considering the various alternative courses open to them to meet what they see as the needs of the patient. Of course they are far from safe against demonic deception but it is not surprising that I am helped by the work of

Christian medical doctors when looking for *methods* of considering the validity of any alternative therapy. We find little help when we look to the alternative practitioners themselves. Dr Andrew Fergusson, a Christian GP, writes that 'orthodox medicine is open to controlled analysis and doctors virtually always change their practice in the light of unfolding truth. Often alternative practitioners are not interested in beginning to examine the basis of their art.' ★

Another doctor, Professor James Payne, who chaired the British Medical Association's Board of Science and Education Working Party on Alternative Medicines which produced a highly critical report looked at more closely in Chapter Eighteen, says "the only philosophy that united the widely divergent therapies was the rejection of the scientific basis of medicine." ★ ★

Dr Keith Sanders, General Secretary of The Christian Medical Fellowship has given doctors a very useful checklist for considering particular therapies. It first appeared in the Christian Medical Fellowship Associates Journal 'Nucleus' (January 1986) and I quote Dr Fergusson's amplification of it in 'Pacemaker', January 1987:

1. Do the claims made for it fit the facts? i.e. so far as it can be tested is it true?

2. Is there a rational scientific basis to the therapy? Medical science is based on a (limited) understanding of God's orderly creation. Does the therapy fit into that framework?

★ Taken from *What's The Alternative?* by Dr Andrew Fergusson (*Pacemaker*, Nurses' Christian Fellowship - January 1987)

★ ★ Quoted in B M A News Review July 1986, p.25

3. Is it the methodology or is it the principle which is the effective element? i.e. if it works, whence does the truth originate?

4. What are the assumptions of the world view behind the therapy? Many alternative medicines are based on Eastern, mystical, Hindu concepts of 'energy' and 'life forces'. Christians will be suspicious of this, but it is possible that good horses can come from bad stables.

5. Does the therapy involve the occult? Is it one of, or like unto, practices specifically forbidden in Scripture? In this context, many practitioners add their own occult elements to therapies which may otherwise be harmless.

6. Has it stood the test of time? This is in general a much weaker test, for although fads and fashions will thereby be eliminated, there are some ancient practices which are questionable ('there's no fool like an old fool').

I believe God would have us use our intellect in the measure that He has given this to us, and throughout the time I have been writing about Alternative Medicine I have been grateful to Christian doctors for bringing to me the reminder that God does not intend that we push our intellect aside when we become aware of the power of His Spirit. As Dr Fergusson has written "the problem of the is-it-true? approach is that truth cannot always be known at the desired time, and we must retain open minds and humble hearts."★ If I were ever to consult a

★ Taken from *What's The Alternative?* by Dr Andrew Fergusson (*Pacemaker,* Nurses' Christian Fellowship - January 1987)

doctor in his surgery I would consider it right to understand as far as possible with my intellect the diagnosis and suggested treatment before asking the Lord if any of it would be against His will. With his checklist, the doctor above is properly taking *his* intellectual approach.

Question one of the checklist is basically concerned with whether the therapy works or not, and whilst that is quite legitimate, it will be seen in a truer perspective as the answers to questions two to five are applied to more and more therapies and become more clear. The rationale of question one is clear when faced with the need to assess a new therapy but we need to emphasise here that it is not in the purpose of this book to concern the reader with whether a therapy works or not. Rather its purpose is to encourage a discernment of the source of its power.

4
A Searcher's Path

One day I was given a peace I had never known. The next day, against incredible odds and without any human planning, I was reunited with a movement called Moral Rearmament (MRA), exactly at the place I had last met with it some twenty years previously.

I had never forgotten MRA's four absolute moral standards (absolute honesty, absolute purity, absolute unselfishness and absolute love) and I had tried to build my life upon them. I had failed and now I saw the answer in fellowship with MRA people. I didn't know that without Jesus I was bound to fail. However I was fired with the idea of 'doing good'! Next came my introduction to spiritual healing. It was all in Satan's plan.

An MRA conference in Switzerland provided the forum for many religions. MRA accommodated me at a Rosicrucian★ hotel. My particular friends there were some distinguished Hindus. Their peace as well as their moral stance greatly attracted me. Unwittingly they had

★ The Rosicrucians are a cult and they believe everything occurs by cosmic, natural law. They tell us that the touch of letters and objects can immediately convey impressions of the sender and of past events. They say the human consciousness can be instantaneously extended out of the body to remote places and events, and that the mental impressions and sight and sound sensations can be communicated at a distance without physical means. They believe thoughts can be changed into things and that we can mentally create useful realities from our ideas. All this is occult. Paracelsus was a Rosicrucian.

41

served an extraordinary purpose in my life and I flew on to my next venue in Scotland for five days of training to become a healer with one of today's outstanding spiritual healers.

By this time I had already been instantaneously 'healed' of haemorrhoids after suffering them for twenty-one years. Little did I realise what the spiritual side-effects of that and my other spiritual involvements would be. Every step I took opened me further to the wiles of Satan. I visited mediums and attended healer training sessions, where I first discovered some of the therapies described in this book. I visited the shrine of Sai Baba, an Indian god-man with counterfeit miracle healing powers. Later I believed I was in communication with his spirit when I received a clear manifestation of his presence. Eventually I prayed to him, and I believed that after my death I would be reincarnated in another body.

Without realising it, I had become a full-time 'searcher'. I read 'The Life of Jesus', a rich red leather edition of 1884 which described Jesus' healing ministry. Also, still as a searcher, I became a regular church attender once again.

In my search I was close to others who were treading the same path. One of these friends became tormented in a dreadful way. I didn't then know about demons; however, he was seeing them. A week later he was found dead. Immediately I went to a Spiritualist Church. Here the medium perfectly described the red leather book to me. 'I have the previous owner with me,' she said. 'Ask your wife. She will know. It is a very important book.' A clever choice of book for the demons to describe! Satan was masquerading as an angel of light. The medium had also described the extraordinary hands of the original owner. I told my wife and she found a snapshot of this old family friend taken some forty years before. The big hands could be seen just as she remembered them.

Previously cool about my search, which was now into its second year, she was at last very interested.

The next day we learned *how* my searcher-friend had died - naked with cuts and bruises. As with the demon-possesed man among the tombs in Mark 5:5, they were self-inflicted. Satan's purpose is to bring death, and this he had done. My wife's interest in searching lasted only twenty-four hours!

After twenty-one months of working on MRA's absolute standards in my life, and as a searcher, I hastily began looking into the dangers. God overruled Satan's intention for my life. By a great miracle I was born again, and God showed me that my healing methods were from Satan.

For twenty years the MRA book *Remaking Men* by Paul Campbell and Peter Howard, had been my 'bible.' As a Christian I renounced my healing involvement; but *not* MRA. Then eventually David Watson wrote this in a letter to me: 'I saw red lights when I read *Remaking Men*, because of the absence of any reference to Christ. Any movement that purports to proclaim Christ must be unashamedly Christ-centred in its writings and proclamations. The very desire to open doors to all faiths is also its definite weakness, and I would not be happy if any Christian got involved in MRA.' Long after I received it, the Lord eventually got through to me by means of that letter. I was set free.

Many, including committed Christians, have turned from drugs to spiritual solutions in the belief that they were natural therapies. I pray the Lord will use the words and Scripture in this book to set more people free.

PART TWO
ALTERNATIVE MEDICINE:
A GUIDE

The witness of the Holy Spirit is vital. Aside from that, we look at either the occult origin (or root) or the nature of any practitioner's involvement contrary to God's word.

In this guide to more than one hundred therapies, it is hoped that Christian readers will be helped to discern themselves whether any particular treatment is of God or not.

Why have I included therapies that are *not* founded in the occult? The answer is that an increasing number of their practitioners are bringing an occult dimension into the therapy. This is a very important point which needs to be kept in mind, and it is particularly true the further we move away from so-called scientific medicine. Perhaps surprisingly, we find less of an intellectual barrier to the utter illogicality of some treatments that are offered. Satan has made his mark on medical science in many ways, including through drugs, but in these days Satan appears to be focusing on alternative therapies subtly designed for an unsuspecting public.

Why then don't I explain each technique? One answer is that I could not do so, even if I believed it would be right. Perhaps one day there will be huge volumes connecting the foundation of, say, reflexology with the systems we see today. But I doubt it! Attempts will be made, but the philosophies often go back more than 5,000 years, and there are new therapies every year.

What can be understood is that nearly all the therapies are in one way or another based upon subtle spiritual implications. Most are derived from the occult, humanistic or religious world views of their originators. This means they stem from a belief system that is contrary to God. In the words of Brooks Alexander of the American research organisation, Spiritual Counterfeits Project: '... the metaphysical framework from which they (the Eastern or occult healing techniques) emerge, is so pervasive and encompasssing that every detail of practice is intricately related to elements of the underlying belief system. As a result the technique taken as a whole will carry overtones and implications of the metaphysical system from which it is derived, even if the system is not explicitly attached.' ★

One of the most often reiterated biblical themes is that we should guard ourselves against deception and separate ourselves from counterfeit spirituality; it is not God's will that we should search for truth among the hidden knowledge. God will give discernment to those who earnestly seek it.

There are two errors in dealing with Satan. One is to deny his existence and power. That is the error of the great majority in these days. The other error is one that we must avoid falling into in the area of alternative medicine; the idea that Satan and his demons are active everywhere and in everything. There is a danger that we can be led into fearing a treatment because Satan *might* be in it — in the therapy or through the therapist. For example, where herbal remedies are concerned, there can be the error of ascribing to Satan something that is from the Lord.

Jesus calls Satan 'the prince (or ruler) of this world'(John 14:30). Satan is the ruler over the affairs of the world and in opposition to God. However the earth is

★ Reprinted by permission of Spiritual Counterfeits Project, Inc. © 1978. PO Box 4308, Berkeley, California 94704, USA 'Holistic Health from the Inside' (*Spiritual Counterfeits Project Journal* - August 1978).

the Lord's and we can confidently use the things that He provides in His creation, giving thanks to Him for them. *'For every creature of God is good, and nothing to be refused, if it be received with thanksgiving: For it is sanctified by the word of God and prayer.'* (1 Timothy 4:4-5). Whilst we should not use any herb or treatment because it has been 'improved ' by magic, and whilst we would not allow treatment by a therapist who, however innocently, was seen to resort to occult power, we are free to use the goodness of the Lord's creation — the plants, the minerals, the animals and all that is in it.

'For God hath not given us the spirit of fear; but of power, and of love, and of a sound mind' (2 Timothy 1:7). Fear is from Satan, and being alert to the wiles of Satan doesn't mean we have to fear him or even pay undue attention to him. Once again, we know that herbal remedies are good and we have the authority of Scripture; therefore unless we get a check in our spirit, or *know* of an occult addition to what God has provided, we are only glorifying Satan when we start to worry or fear.

For therapies where there is some clear occult connection, whether from what is written or from a practitioner's own literature, it will be up to individual Christians to make their decisions. For other therapies, where there is an openness to occult adaptation by the practitioner, Christians can know in their spirits if something is not right; once again the Christian will be free to make a decision. When the Holy Spirit convicts us, we are free to do something about it. Fear however can only be from Satan.

It is true that the mere sight of some therapies (usually the complex or little known ones) mentioned in print in a book like this can lead some to deliverance. In my personal testimony on homoeopathy in Chapter Nine it will be seen that the Lord used a Christian book to start off a long chain of confirmations of the occult basis of homoeopathy. The book hadn't said homoeopathy was occult, but the Holy Spirit did! Taking an example from the First Edition of my own book, one reader, encouraged to scan through the book in the course of deliverance spotted 'chiropractic'.

As she describes in her testimony in Chapter Five, this person received deliverance and healing. Jesus calls driving out demons, 'a miracle' (Mark 9:38-39) and we are seeing more miracles in these days.

Seeing the names of therapies in this book may prompt responses such as the above. Yet in other cases therapies like chiropractic may well produce no response at all from those who have been treated by a chiropractor. Alas, seeing a name might even promote fear! It is no part of my purpose to encourage Satan by referring to therapies in which he is not making any impression! However, it is right, I believe, to include a range of *all* therapies (good and bad) in order to warn that even the best, like physiotherapy, are in these days open to abuse by therapists who, choosing to use occult power, combine other techniques.

The Holy Spirit is the teacher (Luke 12: 12). New therapies are showing themselves all the time. Some are so new that nothing is written about them. Some therapies are backed by doubtful philosophy that the practitioner himself may never have resorted to. It is neither easy nor useful to give more information for all the therapies. However I believe that, perhaps using a check list like the one given in Chapter Ten where necessary, it can be clear which therapies are so clearly occult that discerning Christians will unreservedly reject them. Furthermore in their own situations, where there is a need to know, Christians can hear the answer when they earnestly seek it.

5
So-called physical therapies

The area of so-called 'new' therapies includes **acu-puncture.** The present basis for it was provided by the philosophical school of Taoism founded in the third and fourth centuries B.C. It even dates back 2,000 years before that in ancient China.

Ancestor worship, common in China, has led to sorcery. Their concept of a unity between the universe and man, is common ground with the Hindu and other eastern religions. Thanks in large part to missionary zeal, China now has many Bible-believing Christians. However, undiscerning Christians have brought back much of the demonic that still has not been identified and cast out in the name of Jesus! At one time, acupuncture, used for anaesthesia in China, was refused for the westerners that lived there. It didn't work as well with them! Self-hypnosis and suggestion probably play an important part, and with the faith in acupuncture in the west in these days, anaesthesia by acupuncture on westerners is now said to be working much better.

There are two basic deceptive beliefs: the existence of energy *ch'i* and the presence of invisible energy lines (meridians) that are supposed to direct the energy to all organs of the body. Drawings of different so-called energy lines are to be found in many occult 'healing' techniques. The energy is said to be controlled by the *yin* and the *yang,* two universal opposing yet harmonising forces, which like negative and positive, and male and female permeate all nature. The imbalance of the *yin* and the *yang* is said to hinder the energy flow and cause illness. Practitioners identify some hundreds of acupuncture 'points' along the 'meridian', and they believe that puncture by the needles rebalances the energy and restores health. Although never to be understood, acupuncture is well known today and has been pretty well exposed by Christian writers. Christians have to steer well clear of its occult influence.

Auriculotherapy is a variation of acupuncture, and **acupressure** is rooted in the same philosophy. It involves pressure rather than needles, and so finds favour among the squeamish! Thus it is more acceptable, but equally devastating in its spiritual side-effects. Another energy-balancing therapy, is **moxibustion.** A smouldering fragment of a plant is put on the acupuncture point. The variations can be endless. More creative therapists are into hitting the acupuncture points with laser beams and ultra-sound! A world that has quickly come to accept ideas of meridians and ch'i, readily moves on to more obvious magical practices using the same language. An example is **jin shin do.**

Emile Krémer★ summarises the position the Christian has to take in the following way: 'The origin, nature and development of acupuncture... show clearly that believers dare not expose themselves to the influence of the spirits that have inspired this ancient healing method which is now sweeping through western countries... They are finding the western nations well prepared through all the forms of occultism (superstitions, astrology, witchcraft, etc) which are spreading very rapidly in so-called Christian countries.'

★ *'Eyes Opened to Satan's Subtlety'* by Emile Krémer (M.O.V.E. Press - 1969)

Christians need to be aware of the activities of cults and of occult practices apart from occult healing therapies, in order to counsel others and take a clear stand as witness to the truth found in God's word. The Bible tells us, *'Even him, whose coming is after the working of Satan with all power and signs and lying wonders, and with all deceivableness of unrighteousness in them that perish; because they received not the love of the truth, that they might be saved.'* (2 Thess. 2:9-10).

The whole range of occult therapies includes many that overlap one with another. There are obvious overlaps, too, with the cults and other occult practices. Satan doesn't arrange his wiles in tidy compartments and there is no way that language can adequately describe this spiritual realm. Chapter Ten contains a list of areas that may be helpful in Christian counselling, in order to identify occult involvement. Some understanding of a therapy or occult involvement will often be desirable and I have, I believe, written more than enough about acupuncture in this and previous pages, to establish the status it must have with Christians. An undue interest in the detail is often far from desirable. It is the 'Way Out that is most important! This is through *renunciation* of the therapy, *repentance* of involvement with it, and *faith in Jesus Christ and His atoning blood.* The help of other Christians may also be needed by those who are deeply affected, in order that the powers of Satan can be rebuked, and healing and deliverance brought to them in the name of Jesus.

Once again, **reflexology** is traceable back to China 5,000 years ago. It was also known in ancient Egypt. Practitioners believe there are ten energy channels, each covering all the organs in a zone of the body. By feeling the feet they believe they can find which channel is blocked; then they massage the feet seeking to restore the energy flow. I have studied and done this myself. There has perhaps been little detailed research into the orgins, beyond what millions are reading in modern-day 'alternative health' guides. There is enough for the discerning Christian!

Again along similar lines, and perhaps originating in Europe, there is **polarity therapy.** Away from Taoism and China now, it is necessary to look for other clues to the occult root. Its founder made an extensive study of eastern medicine and his spiritual inspiration came from India. Polarity therapists believe there are five centres in the body (the etheric, the air, the fire, the water and the earth) and that they need to be balanced in order for the energy to flow. The energy charts are once again different. Is it not deception?

The question for the intellect is: What, if any, is the scientific basis for these ideas? And, if there is none, from what spiritual kingdom do they come? They are not like electric current — unseen, difficult to understand, but understood by the scientist. They belong to the spiritual dimension.

Yoga is not merely a physical therapy. All those who practise it come under the influence of its occult powers. This is so whether or not there is any awareness of its Hindu origin and whether or not it is the intention not 'to go too far!' It is very dangerous.

I practised yoga myself. However it wasn't until researching more detail for this book that I discovered the true extent of yoga's influence in Britain. I was put in touch with an organisation called 'Friends of Yoga', a branch of an Indian registered trust.

The Vice-President of Friends of Yoga wrote to me: 'Yoga is *not* a religion, but all religions have their roots in yoga philosophy, including Christianity.' She wrote, 'Christ himself was one of the greatest Bhakti/Karma yogis that ever lived. The Surya Namaskar (Salute to the Sun) can be done to the Lord's Prayer, and I learned it this way from a Catholic missionary, who is himself a devoted Christian and a practising yogi.'

The truth is that yoga aims to liberate us from the normal human condition and to replace this with a 'higher state of consciousness' in which man can see himself as divine. There is nothing Christian about it. Yoga can never be safe. It can affect body and soul, as well as bringing eternal danger to the spirit. It aims to let the supposed 'latent element' or 'true self' within man shine out as god. It is a counterfeit.

We don't easily learn the lessons of Adam and Eve and the fall of man. *'And the serpent said unto the woman, ye shall not surely die: For God doth know that in the day ye eat thereof, then your eyes shall be opened, and ye shall be as gods, knowing good and evil.'* (Genesis 3:4-5). It was Satan's lie. The truth is in God's word. The Holy Spirit living in those who know Jesus as Saviour and Lord is quite different from the yoga idea of man being divine. There is no latent element in man; we are nothing until we receive Jesus. *'But as many as received him, to them gave he power to become the sons of God, even to them that believe on his name.'* (John 1:12).

Hinduism is the prevailing world view in the west today and every yoga teacher can be seen as a Hindu or Buddhist missionary. Christianity is quickly and progressively being eliminated from western schools, and the emphasis is shifting to teaching about other people's religions. This is overtly done and it supports the Hindu and eastern deceptions that prevail in alternative medicine, the cults, all of the occult and the New Age movement we look at in Chapter Twelve.

Those practising yoga don't discover their 'true self'. Rather they progressively open themselves up, through their passivity, to invasion by demons. Sometimes they use a mantra, a name of a Hindu god given to enable contact with him by calling his name or mantra. Of course contact is with the Satanic realm, and I used the mantra *om*. Once the demons take over, they are viewed as the 'god within'.

If those who practise yoga and don't know Jesus, will take the step of faith, repent, and ask Jesus to come into their lives, they will be born again and they will become new creations. They will have the Holy Spirit dwelling within them. Only then will yoga practitioners know that what they had before was a counterfeit peace, and that the thief had come only to kill and steal and destroy. Jesus is the one that brings life, and with Him they can have it to the full. (John 10:10).

Again from China, there is **t'ai chi**. As the name suggests, the aim is to tune into the 'ch'i' energy. It seems to be a sort of civilian martial art. Martial arts are an expression of eastern spiritual philosophy. The body is said to have an intrinsic energy, ch'i, which can be developed by special techniques. Faith in this ch'i soon comes to those that participate. Satan is the the author of the supernatural powers seen in martial arts; they are *not* energies dormant within us. From India there is Indian Boxing (not very common). From China; Ch'uan-fa or Kung-Fu. From Korea there is Taekwondo. The best known are Judo and Karate; along with many others, they come from Japan.

To the onlooker T'ai Chi looks like a spiritual dance. One practitioner saw it, not only as a means to combat the illnesses of mind and body but as a way of understanding the 'inner nature'. However the understanding that results is that of Tao philosophy. Although T'ai Chi is much older in concept, it is said that the philosophy of T'ai Chi developed from the more elementary idea of defence around the twelfth century.

T'ai Chi means the underlying unity of all manifestation and it is designed to integrate the personality with the spirit by alignment of energies and the opening up of what are seen as higher faculties. In other words practitioners are coming deeper into the Satanic realm, the counterfeit of Christians who receive more light as they walk with Jesus.

54

It is once again emphasised that the explanation of t'ai chi, yoga, acupuncture, or any of these deceptions, is nothing more than an attempt at some description of the process to the so-called peace, healing and eventual enlightenment that the underlying philosophies promise. The description is as the deceived will see it. The explanations of ch'i, yin, yang, and the endless diagrams that appear in the catalogues and prospectuses of the promoters, are nothing but deception. On first view of such literature Christians may conclude that people must be crazy to fall for it! However Satan has a powerful foothold with many in these days.

From Japan, there is **aikido,** a so-called exercise or movement therapy along the lines of T'ai Chi. These so-called 'soft' or 'internal' martial arts include also a form of karate known as **mushindo karate.** Compared to the 'hard' martial arts described previously, they are much more concerned with mental discipline, meditation and submission to occult power. Thus, and not surprisingly to those who have some awareness of Satan's schemes, it is these gentle drawing room martial arts that are the really powerful ones. These 'soft' varieties are especially dangerous and subtle, but this should not in any way minimise the occult dangers in those more familiar ones that have a spectacular and vigorous element.

Again from Japan, there is **shiatsu** which seems to be akin to acupressure. Shiatsu has been a traditional occupation for the blind in Japan, and now we have seen a course introducing Shiatsu to the Blind in Britain at a Tibetan Buddist Retreat in Cumbria. The Royal National Institute for the Blind (RNIB) inform me: 'With the present general interest in alternative medicine it is natural that several enquiries have been made by visually handicapped persons interested in Shaitsu as a possible career.' The RNIB runs the North London School of Physiotherapy where visually handicapped students are prepared for the examinations of the Chartered Society of Physiotherapy, and the unsighted are in many ways especially suited to this sort of work. It is a tragedy to find the inroads shiatsu is making into this much respected body of unsighted people.

I identify all of the foregoing therapies as ones that Christians will want to avoid. And there are dozens more. What about Rudolf Steiner's **anthroposophical medicine?** Like homoeopathy this is accommodated by the medical profession in Britain. It seems to be a mixture of occult concepts and it is allied to homoeopathy. The first therapeutic centre of its kind in the English-speaking world, offering residential anthroposophical treatment, was opened recently close to my own home.

The origins of **Bach flower remedies** seem also to present a clear case. They consist of 38 remedies prepared from flowers on a formula devised by Dr Edward Bach. They treat negative states of mind which he believed were the causes of any disorder. So far so good! But further enquiry shows that Bach was a diviner. He found that by holding his hand over a flowering plant, if for example he was despondent, it enabled him to find the plant to cure his despondency. The distance Christians put between themselves and Bach remedies (and indeed all of these methods) will be something they have to decide for themselves.

It is true that some of today's orthodox medicine may be rooted in the occult. Where do you draw the line? Only God can answer individuals on that. Orthodox medicine, with modern drugs, has advanced to the stage where investigation of all its occult roots would be very difficult. The symbol of the British Medical Association includes the serpent!

It may be that some **herbal concoctions** would be appropriate subjects for research. Of course the simple herbs, used in their own right since Bible times, have a

God-given healing quality. '... *and the fruit thereof shall be for meat, and the leaf thereof for medicine'* (Ezekiel 47:12). However further enquiry is worthwhile where herbal mixtures are founded in magic, where formulae are given by divination, or where herbs are collected as charms are recited. As with orthodox medicine, no sweeping generalisations can be made.

Nicholas Culpepper (1616-1654) was perhaps the most famous of the traditional herbalists. He trained as an apothecary (the forerunner of the GP today). Then he went on in what he believed to be science, combining herbalism with astrology. Astrology is the occult art of deriving knowledge from the stars and their influence on, in Culpeppers's case, plant life. In its origin and nature, astrology is idolatrous and Satanic; and so what of the origins of some of the concoctions that Culpepper formulated?

More herbal remedies are today becoming available from the east. **Ginseng,** regarded by the Chinese as a cure-all and a 'gift from the gods' has been heavily promoted.

The Chinese and Koreans have used ginseng for over 5,000 years. I mention this herb specifically because it is so highly regarded in the East. What can be said about it? One booklet used for sales promotion tells us the orientals regarded the shape of the root (it closely resembles a human body) as a sign from the powers that be that this was the herb for man. I read that it took six years for it to grow and that a great deal of ceremony surrounds both the planting and the harvesting. It seems there are quality grades. The first is 'Heaven' or 'King', the second grade is 'Earth' and the third is 'Good' or 'Man'. I read that 'vast' research has gone into ginseng since 1854! In conclusion, somewhat suprisingly, I read, '... neither is there any evidence that ginseng is able to cure any specific ailment.' Whatever the strange conclusion of this particular sales promotion pamphlet, I don't doubt that hundreds have put their faith in ginseng and seen their symptoms disappear. Needless to say, that is not the point. What of the **hakims** (or 'Wise Men'), the relatively new arrivals from the Indian subcontinent dispensing native herbalism?

The manipulation that is the essential feature of **osteopathy** and **chiropractic** may appear to be well founded. However since osteopathy is illegal in countries like Belgium, closer enquiry into these major therapies may well be timely.

These are days of variety with alternative medicine practitioners, ignorant of the spiritual aspects, looking in on one another's methods. Also quite apart from the non-Christian philosophies in which the therapies are rooted, the nature of the treatments given by the osteopath and chiropractor, using the hands almost throughout, leaves any misguided practitioner well open to what Satan is up to in these days. Whilst a 'searcher' in the occult realm of medicine I received training from such a practitioner.

Chiropractic may well be sound as a therapy for spine adjustment, but its practitioners move to dangerous ground when they swallow the energy ideas. Palmer, the founder, identified an energy which he called the 'innate' and he believed its flow through the nervous system could be blocked by spinal misalignments. Osteopathy works on various levels, according to one health guide, and Still, its founder, was, like the acupuncturists, thinking of other body healing forces.

Naturopathy, involving diet, fasting and exercise, can once again be helpful to good health. However this innocent-sounding therapy has come to mean something more than a package of natural treatments. One natural health clinic describes naturopathy very fairly as a holistic approach combining multiple methods best suited to the individual and including the use of diet, fasting, exercises and structural adjustments. However the reality in the centres that are proliferating in these days is that the 'multiple methods' will usually include at least one occult treatment method. Few are alert to the dangers.

Christians are more and more open to the accusation: '... but you are condemning nearly everything.' That reality only reflects the depths to which health care has so very recently, and so very quickly, fallen.

Touch for health is born out of chiropractic and ancient eastern knowledge, and is another approach that combines a number of methods. Many of these therapies will understandably involve the counterfeit of the biblical laying-on-of-hands and another is the **Reiki programme.** The idea is that we lay hands and tap a higher frequency of powerful cosmic healing energy. **Biopathy** is yet another synthesis of ancient and modern wisdom, and anyone joining the programme could well meet reflexology, Bach flower remedies, acupuncture, and much else besides. What about **Massage?** Of course this can be a legitimate physical therapy. Contrary to that fact, Holistic Healing practitioners see massage as a 'healing art,' and in 'The Massage Book'★ which has sold more than three quarters of a million copies, we find that definition confirmed. And for a description of the massage we read that a person normally falls into a mental-physical state 'difficult to describe.' It is likened to going into a hidden and unfamiliar room, the existence of which is only to be recognised by those practising some form of daily meditation. What we have there is a good description of an altered state of consciousness. These so-called physical therapies, following the New Agers' own definition, are in fact part of Satan's battle for the Mind, a 'transformation of consciousness' throughout society. Society is being conditioned to

★ 'The Massage Book' by G Downing (Random House, New York - 1984)

accept the occult as quite normal. We look at Mind Control techniques under the heading of 'So-Called Psychological Therapies' in the next chapter, and it is through this 'new consciousness' 'cosmic consciousness', 'transformation of consciousness' or 'awareness' that minds are brought under the control of demons and called 'spirit guides'. We shall see that children, to be relieved of stress, are encouraged to contact 'wise men' in 'Quieting Reflex' therapy, and cancer sufferers are to contact their 'inner guides' in 'Guided Imagery' therapy. The next chapter deals also with Mind Control techniques of various kinds. We shall see that deception attends the idea that the mind can cause disease. Yet Satan can reach his goal via our bodies and Massage, a physical therapy at the hands of a Holistic Healer, is the start of a journey, via our minds into Satan's realm.

And in all these therapies, it's the *practice* we have to identify. Names can vary. Massage is sometimes called **Bodywork.**

In these days we can no longer ignore the spiritual status of those who treat us; nevertheless it is emphasised again and again in this book that the mere mention of an alternative treatment is not to be taken as any suggestion that it should necessarily be avoided. However, Christians will want to approach all with caution. Among the best established and admirable of the therapies is **physiotherapy.** The Chartered Society of Phsyiotherapy, in a position paper submitted to the BMA in December 1983, considered many so-called 'alternative' techniques were already available from the physiotherapist within orthodox medical care. The paper acknowledged its interest in recognisable alternatives. I believe the floodgates are open, and the Society should note that many of these alternatives are not what they seem.

The paper makes it clear that the Society has no definition of physiotherapy, 'preferring the term to remain flexible because too rigid a definition would have the effect of imposing potentially restrictive boundaries on the further development of a still growing profession.' The following assessment of the profession by the Chartered Society provides a realistic view of the way it is set to make its contribution to the quiet revolution that is taking place in health care: 'There is now a greater understanding of the significance of the deliberate professional use of touch by chartered physiotherapists and their use of highly skilled manipulative techniques, and of the effectiveness of touch as a means of healing.' There is now a greater understanding of the effectiveness of touch as a means of sensory input and emotional contact and its implications for 'healing'! Physiotherapists must not go too far. The Society has a strong commitment to research in physiotheraphy and to developing further the research base, but it needs to know that a loving touch is one thing, and the 'deliberate professional use of touch' for 'healing' can be quite another. It leads to therapy along the lines of therapeutic touch and the paranormal spiritual therapies, which are not from God, and which are looked at in Chapter Seven.

The following is taken from the testimony of Janice, a young Christian woman who, in pain and desperation, went to a physiotherapist who was 'highly recommended' by her friends:

'I was born with legs of slightly uneven length. When I was at university, and in desperation to get back on my feet after a 'slipped disc', I visited a physiotherapist. He said he had improved on his physiotherapy treatments through a study of Chinese medicine. He told me how he had overcome paralysis as a boy by sheer will power. I had not then come into the revelation of Jesus' power to heal today, but as I was told more and more of his medical beliefs, I became increasingly worried. On my final visit he held my feet and told me he could learn about the health of the body through doing this. He told me I had had kidney trouble in the past. He was right, for I had kidney stones when I was sixteen. Then he said that when he was massaging a back he could always tell if a person had cancer because he felt something like thick green sludge, and "they" would tell him he could no longer treat the person. Who "they" were, I dreaded to ask! He said he could tell where the pain centres were as he only had to run his hand over my back, two or three inches over my skin, and electric shock went from his hand to the spot. Again he was quite right, and I used to feel it. Finally he told me he practised "astral projection"★ and that he could stop and restart his heart at will... As I had not come into correct teaching I didn't listen to the promptings of the Spirit early enough.

'I repented of my involvement with this physiotherapist... Interestingly, he could never get my back right although I know he never had any problems with a lot of other peoples'! Now I knew he was not only a physiotherapist, but also a spiritualist, a healer and a reflexologist.

'About two years ago my back was badly injured when I lifted some very heavy files at work. My doctor, and a surgeon, said this time the injury was so bad the only thing that could help was surgery, but the chances of success were only fifty-fifty. I was bedridden and in agony, but I was not prepared to take those odds... However, John, my husband, and I were not quite sure how to pray and so to "buy time" and to get the surgeon "off my back"while I studied the Scriptures and found someone who believed in divine healing and who would pray in faith, we decided I should undergo some manipulative treatment. I was careful to avoid obvious satanic workers in alternative medicine in choosing

★ Astral projection is an occult experience which involves leaving the body.

someone to provide treatment, but I did not yet realise there were dangers in "respectable" alternative medicine too.

'One of the elders in our church was visiting a chiropractor and another friend had recently had her back put right by a chiropractor. After four months totally bedridden I began to receive chiropractic treatment. After an initial visit for diagnosis, the chiropractor explained the damage. This is where I think practitioners in alternative medicine especially succeed. They are kind and show understanding to the patient. They explain everything and unlike so many NHS situations they have time to make you feel you matter, which is so very important. The chiropractor explained that I had a cracked vertebra, advanced spondylitis, a twisted pelvis and sacrum, and uneven leg lengths. Six weeks after the treatment began, my pelvis was eventually straightened, but soon it twisted again. John and I were trusting more and more in the Lord for healing and we had twice received instantaneous improvement after praying in faith. However we were still relying on the chiropractor too. Alternative medicine has an insidious draw.

'After six months we took a slow and painful trip to spend a week away. We made the journey equipped with x-rays and the name of a local chiropractor. I needed his "patch up" treatment for the return journey. He told me it was likely I would be crippled by the age of thirty-five. I was then twenty-four. John and I were very depressed. On the journey home the Lord challenged us: "Will you believe this chiropractor's prognosis or will you believe my promise to heal?" It was hard but we knew the Lord was right and we decided to believe Him and not the chiropractor's prognosis. My condition then deteriorated for three weeks! However we pressed into our faith and proclaimed our trust in the Lord.

'At the end of the three weeks we heard of a healing meeting at a local renewal gathering and we asked the

Lord if I should go. He marvellously confirmed that I should go and that He would heal me. At the end of the meeting an evangelist prayed with me in Jesus' name. The power of God so flooded through me that it set all my bones into place. It shortened my longer leg as well. I had received my healing.

'Three days later I was due to visit the chiropractor. I had no need of more treatment but wished to show him just what had happened. He was utterly astounded. He was edgy and nervous but had to accept the evidence before him. He confirmed that everything was in place. My doctor too, confirmed that I was healed.

'Although I had finished with the chiropractor, the effects of the treatment with both him and the physiotherapist had not ended in the spiritual realm. Many weeks after I was healed, I suddenly started getting severe sciatica. I realised this was a satanic attack but was not aware of the reason. I contacted two Christians whom the evangelist recommended, and their discernment was that I needed to be cut off from the effect of the physiotherapist and to receive deliverance. The sciatica left. However I was now receiving a pain in my hip. This seemed like a mirror of what I had once felt there, but not quite like the real thing. They gave me *Beware Alternative Medicine* ★ to read to see if it might jog my memory of any other thing in my past. They knew about the chiropractor but were unsure if that was the cause.

'I began reading Roy Livesey's exposé following the directions for protection by the blood of Jesus. When I got to the section which mentioned chiropractic, I felt something in me leap into my throat and almost a shriek or most urgent whisper in my ear, "No, not that!" I then

★ *Beware Alternative Medicine* by Roy Livesey was the First Edition of this book. The title of the Second Edition was changed to 'Understanding Alternative Medicine.'

realised that the suspicions expressed in the book were correct, and that I needed further prayer for deliverance. We called it a "Spirit of Chiropractice" and my friends commanded it to leave in the name of Jesus. The spirit went, and the pain in my hip left with it.

'That was a year ago. I am fit and active, horse riding again and lifting heavy toddlers and babies without trouble and with great joy and praise for His wonderful name.'

Much illness is certainly caused by the way man uses his body and the **Alexander method** aims at personal freedom and health through a voluntarily applied discipline. Then there is **breathing therapy, air therapy** and **earth therapy.** Therapies are not necessarily as innocuous as they sound, and these have their place with others in the typical alternative health guide helping to blur the identity of other innocuous-sounding therapies which are either rooted in the occult or from a false religious basis. Breathing! We can usually do that safely enough, but not always. There is a therapy called **holonomic integration breathing** where various techniques from eastern and western psycho-therapies, bodywork, cultural and spiritual traditions, can be used. Alternatively there is a healing technique mysteriously described as **rebirthing.** One leaflet describes this as a powerful yet gentle healing method which gives you 'an experience of mastery' in your life. The deep breathing is to enable you to take on board new thoughts that empower you while at the same time letting go of the old thoughts.

Schussler's **tissue salts therapy** reckons body cells can absorb essential salts in small (homoeopathic) doses. As a follower of Hahnemann's homoeopathic methods, his biochemistry involves an occult element. One therapy that appears to be free of the occult is **ionisation therapy.** We are told a concentration of positive ions in the atmosphere is bad for health. Where the therapist sees the need, there is equipment to produce negative ions.

A good rule is to know the spiritual status of the therapist. By listing **dance therapy, art therapy** and **music therapy,** it is easy to appear extreme. The difficulty is with words. No-one will deny that dancing, art and music can be properly therapeutic. There can be sound common sense, but beware psychological excursions linked to these organised therapies. An example is the 'guided imagery', aided by music, that is looked at in Chapter Six. One therapist tells us that cosmic man is like a butterfly emerging from its chrysalis and that his sensitivity has 'not just to be experienced but also to be understood'. We are invited to let ourselves be opened up to the 'subtle worlds of colour and sound.' Indeed we do agree, things are not always what they seem. More and more common are subliminal cassette tapes. One catalogue of 'Peaceful New Age Music' tells us, 'You hear only the music, while absorbing and acting upon the subliminal messages.' What of other relaxing music that the promoters describe as New Age, and induce states of 'inner attunement' and 'healing'? The spiritually blind are coming into the spiritual counterfeits that abound in these days. What is offered *is* attractive. We are in a stressed society and we *do* need to relax. Satan is only too willing to help in this; then he will lead the unaware beyond their expectations. There is no other way but to seek the discernment that is available to those who know Jesus.

Satan knows no boundaries, no neat divisions between one alternative therapy and another, and no careful distinction between a cure and a cosmetic. His purpose is to bring spiritual death. One merchant of so-called **holistic cosmetics** tells us that the human aura seen by clairvoyants and healers as coloured rays comes from the 'vital force' stored in our bodies. The moisturising body oil that is used is said to help restore the balance of body energies.

What about **Bates eyesight training?** Here there is emphasis on the importance of the imagination as an aid to better vision. Faced with a bewildering expansion of alternative treatments Christians will need to take their own view. **Sound therapists** have the idea that every organ has its own frequency of vibration which can be altered by sound waves to produce healing. Are they not blinded by science? *'Professing themselves to be wise, they became fools.'* (Romans 1:22).

Hydrotherapy, the taking of pure spa water, is no doubt harmless to some and valuable to many. The Lord provides this spa water and it is 'good'. What of **aromatherapy,** whether involving herbal medicine at one level or as a relaxing beauty therapy at another? **Macrobiotics** is, on the face of it, selection of diet, but in truth it is a system of choosing food, from Japan, and governed by the principles of yin and yang. A Christian doctor writes 'medically it can be very dangerous, especially for children.' It is an intuitive way of living to remain healthy; it is not the Christian way.

Massage and bodywork therapies often have a religious base and claim to correct energy imbalances. In **zone therapy,** and as we have seen in acupuncture and reflexology, manipulation in certain zones of surface anatomy is said to have a creative effect on some distant organ. However, once again there is no known neurological pathway. In **orgonomy (Reichian therapy),** the energy is called 'orgone energy', derived from 'orgasm'. Reich believed this energy could be released by uninhibited sexual activity. **Bio-energetics** is a method that involves active and passive exercises. It stresses the body in unfamiliar ways and is a sort of psychotherapy to deal with stress. In **do-in,** the practitioner calls the energy 'universal energy' and he uses massage techniques, rather than needles or anything else, to get a good energy flow. The **Feldenkrais technique** involves 'functional integration'! It uses physical and meditative exercises derived from yoga. **Rolfing** (or 'structural integration') is a method to get correct posture and relieve energy blockages. The patient is subjected to physical pressure, and emotional release is said to occur.

In Britain, therapists enjoy a freedom. New therapists, often with variations on the old therapies, are appearing all the time. There is a greater involvement in all kinds of cult and occult activity, and a selection is listed in Chapter Ten. As a result of this activity the world is made more open to deception by these therapies. Christians should understand that most of these therapists are well meaning and sincere. '... *we wrestle not against flesh and blood';* but against the powers of darkness. (Ephesians 6:12). The therapists are deceived by the powers of darkness but they are clear and positive in their objective to bring physical healing. It is no part of their purpose deliberately to deceive Christians. Their literature can be freely read, and they are invariably generous in their explanations of what they seek to do.

The therapies are the spiritual counterfeits to divine healing and as such it is not surprising that most of the therapies are very simple. It is said of the great yogis that when they achieved what they saw as godhood, still they were not satisified and had to build philosophies around themselves. It is the same with new therapists today. Their philosophies and explanations are not new, and neither were those of the yogis before them.

Christians will often find it easy to assess a therapy or therapist on the basis either of what is said or of what is committed to print in leaflets, catalogues, etc. We can look at a therapy as far as we can for ourselves, then when we need to, we can trust God to speak into the situation where we are uncertain.

God made us in such a way that very often healing will naturally take place without human effort. That, I suggest, is not the 'natural' healing that many ascribe to the therapies I am describing. These therapies usually involve faith, and faith involves a choice between the truth and a lie.

Christians know that the ultimate truth behind all creation is God himself. We put our faith in Him, and that faith '... *cometh by hearing, and hearing by the word of God.*' (Romans 10:17). Every area of knowledge that man explores apart from God ends up as a faith system, and in any case man is a reasoning creature who will inevitably put his faith in something.

The faith that is purely in the mind, as distinct from the God-kind of faith which is in the spirit and based upon a sound relationship with Him, is an unsound faith. Many therapies draw upon this sort of faith whatever other occult character they may have.

The idea of energy is at the root of much of alternative medicine. But what of demons? This so-called energy is what some religions have called God or the 'force.' We are told we are entering a New Age and it is assumed that the increasing scientific research into the paranormal will validate the ideas of this energy and bring a marriage of science and what is being called the New Age movement (the new religion).

While British universities begin to follow the patterns seen in America with research into parapsychology, believing it can be a scientific study, centres are opening up at grass roots level to harness the energy that some academics are only now starting to look at. In one such British New Age Centre, the aim is to bring people together in an atmosphere of harmony and caring, 'to help find a balance within and thus create a greater quality of life for themselves.' They run different workshops. For example in the Crystal Workshop New Agers can experience 'different crystals, flows and energies.'

They can learn 'about crystals past and present' and they can 'transform' through crystal meditation and healing! For the more technically minded there are classes and clinics on **mora therapy.** Its proponents expect it to become the medicine of the twenty-first century.

Away from the practitioners themselves and the understanding of energy they are receiving, whether from crystal or from electromagnetic medicine, universities are for the first time taking a real interest. In December 1984 Edinburgh University invited applications for its first Professor of Parapsychology. The press release from the university told us that the Koestler Chair of Parapsychology would be the first such established professorial post in Britain. It is now established and is part of the Faculty of Social Sciences, and the staff of the internationally-known Department of Psychology, in which the new professor is located, were said to have unanimously expressed the wish to have the new chair in their department.

The terms of the £500,000 endowment bequest stipulate that the word 'parapsychology' is to be understood to mean the scientific study of 'paranormal phenomena' in particular the capacity attributed to some individuals 'to interact with their environment by means other than the recognised sensory and motor channels.'

Perhaps the new research at Edinburgh will include a study of ley-lines. Occultists believe that ley-lines carry energy in the earth and give it out to people and other life on the planet. I have myself spent time on the Scottish hillsides with my pendulum looking for these ley-lines! Then there is the energy that some believe influences the water diviner's rod; many a churchgoer is blind to the evil of water diving, and of course these things *do* work. The psychic healer is said to transfer energy to his patient. Demons are at work in all these areas. Then there are the energy-balancers we have looked at in this section of the alternative medicine guide. We are said to be energy around which matter is built. What we can see is supposedly not the reality; reality is found only through our 'higher self'! Although this is a false idea, it is demonstrable when consciousness is altered. It is the thinking prominent in eastern religions.

Experiences in altered states of consciousness through meditation, drugs, and these energy ideas, give rise to the idea that 'all is one'. Admittedly it is difficult for the mind to comprehend this sort of language describing occult experiences. One evening as a 'searcher' I spent many hours with a spiritualist medium. 'I am at one with that vase,' she told me, as she pointed to the porcelain on the mantle shelf. Slowly I came to understand her 'all is one' situation. The distinctions we recognise had disappeared for her. Another result of this new consciousness is the disappearance of the distinction between good and evil. New Age people aim to become aware of this divine nature, and against all that the Bible teaches. Their enlightenment, altered consciousness and experiences of spiritual power serve to show them they have succeeded.

Today many scientists are caught up in the occult explosion and their findings have to be increasingly regarded with great caution and discernment. Happily those scientists who are *not* caught up in it will not take these so-called energies very seriously.

New Age healing looks not to God or to medical science, but to energies, forces, radiations, vibrations and the equivalent word in every false religion or occult therapy. The gospel of the New Age may be reduced to Satan's lies as given to Adam and Eve, 'You will be like God, and you will not die.' This idea of man as a divine being is being promoted in alternative medicine; Satan would subtly draw us from the idea of worshipping our Creator.

We are all in God's plan. We are known to Him as individuals . It is that way with Satan too. It makes little difference to Satan or to the patient if a well-meaning acupuncturist with his heart in the right place puts his needles in the wrong place. It makes no difference, and that is one of the ways new techniques are born! There are new ones all the time. One is **orthobionomy.** I received an impressive-looking certificate with a seal and a Californian name on it. My training lasted two days. With Satan on my side I didn't need even one day! It worked! I didn't know it but I was part of New Age medicine.

We have set down the 'So-Called Physical Therapies' in advance of the 'So-Called Psychological Therapies' described in the chapter following. This is a logical sequence because Satan wants control of our minds and he seeks to achieve that also through our bodies. Most so-called physical therapies lead in this direction. The evil one achieves his same purposes through other branches of the occult and the New Age movement, and through many of the pagan religions and cults. 'Gods of the New Age' ★ is the title of an important Christian film exposing live the present day cult activity. Bhagwan Shree Rajneesh might be better known in the popular press in Britain for his ownership of dozens of Rolls Royce automobiles. Yet, until he was recently driven from America by the authorities, he was the leader of a

★   This is a full length film available on video. 'Filmed on three continents, the film explains why 60 million Americans have exchanged the certain hope of salvation for the hopeless cycle of reincarnation. Why thousands of churchgoers have begun to believe the lies first told by the serpent in the Garden of Eden. Why yoga, meditation, psychological therapy and self-help are turning millions to a pagan worldview, while being taught in our seminaries, churches and schoolrooms.''

Available in the U K on VHS for sale or hire from Christian Information Outreach, 92 The Street, Boughton, Faversham, Kent ME13 9AP.

powerful cult. The film shows the disciples singing of their love for him, with drums beating faster and faster. People are almost frantic by the time the drum stops. This sort of extreme physical activity, best recognised by most of us in the frantic scenes at many a disco, is one way into passivity. Satan has many physical ways that lead to passivity. He can empty our minds through yoga or through massage, through the drum beats or through the disco. Then the empty mind is available to him.

6
So-called psychological therapies

Foremost in the field of these therapies is **hypnotherapy**. This uses **hypnosis** which is increasingly accepted in the medical profession. Christians today are almost generally agreed that hypnotism opens the way for evil spirits. Indeed Emile Krémer has described it as the most effective way. His book *Eyes Opened to Satan's Subtlety* printed in seven languages, has the following to say about hypnosis:

> Serious damage to the soul is thereby done, quite apart from the fact that the patient's spirit is bound by hypnotic, spiritistic and occult powers. This ancient oriental art of suggestion and hypnotism, which is of demonic origin and has been used in magic and divination by the most ancient nations, has reappeared under the seemingly innocent cloak of 'modern science' and paves the way for similar modern methods of 'healing' and delusion. Through the complete elimination of will-power and of the conscious use of the senses, hypnotism is the most effective way of opening the door to all sorts of evil spirits.

Readily available, in some Health Food stores and advertised in many places, we find **self-hypnosis tapes** for use in our own cassette recorders. Favoured by large numbers who would not yet venture to a hypnotist, they are very dangerous. Let eyes be opened to Satan's subtlety! Once again we see the introduction of subliminal sounds to bring what the merchants describe as 'a brilliant new concept in self-improvement and healing.' Freud reckoned our subconscious controlled most of our lives. The customers want their lives changed in one way or another; the subliminal tapes, reaching into the subconscious seem to provide the answer the easy way. All that the conscious hears is the sound of the ocean or the singing of birds!

"The thief cometh not, but for to steal, and to kill, and to destroy: I am come that they might have life, and that they might have it more abundantly." (John 10:10). Satan wants us in a passive state whether this is achieved through yoga, hypnosis or any other way. When we abandon ourselves in these ways, Satan is given an opportunity. He is a legalist and his demons are given a right to oppress us. The particular technical method is less important than grasping the principle involved.

Another method is **meditation.** When proficient, no help will be needed from another in order to 'switch off'. What we are describing here is the counterfeit of Christian meditation, which is quite a different thing. Meditation has been made well known by the Beatles. They innocently provided the publicity for **transcendental meditation** which is now a multi-million dollar business. The effect of meditation is that the mind is emptied or concentrated on something other than the mind of God. It is opened up and demons take over. Meditation goes beyond the thinking mind. It transcends it. Today there are aids of every description - from mantras to monitoring devices - to speed meditators to higher levels of consciousness.

For me, sophisticated electroencephalograph (EEG) machines were used to encourage my progress to alpha brainwave patterns and higher meditation states. Transcendental Meditation, or *TM* as it is most commonly called, is very dangerous. For the Beatles, wasn't it the next step after the drug scene, and do we not see a parallel in medicine today? It was reported in May 1984 that there were doctors at one hospital who were persuading patients that peace of mind through TM might be a better cure for their ills than their pills. It was argued that putting TM on prescription, and making it free under the National Health Service, could save hundreds of millions of pounds. It may not be long before the politicians see the economic possibilities in such a proposition!

It is claimed that some 130,000 practise TM in Britain. A growing number of doctors use it themselves and recommend it for patients. Several hundred have formed an association to campaign for TM to be made available under the NHS. For these reasons and more it was encouraging to see the tests, quoted previously from Dr Keith Sanders and based on the work of Christian Szurko, applied in another article in 'Pacemaker' to Transcendental Meditation. The answers to the six questions present a useful study. They are reproduced in full with the doctor's conclusion:

1. Do the claims made for it fit the facts?

Although much has been claimed for TM which is not open to objective testing, there is evidence published in reputable journals such as The Lancet and the B M J (by, for example, Dr Patel, a GP in Croydon) that TM does at a scientifically acceptable level produce measurable and beneficial physiological changes such as a reduced heart rate, reduced respiratory rate, decreased oxygen consumption, decreased blood pressure, changes in skin resistance suggesting relaxation, changes in alpha-activity in the EEG, and reduction in blood lactate levels. At a simple clinical level, TM can thus help stress and hypertension, for example.

2. Is there a rational scientific basis to the therapy?

The facts above speak for themselves. The mind controls much of the bodily function; relax the mind and the body must benefit. It is doubtful that a Christian who was a scientist could object here.

3. Is it the methodology or is it the principle which is the effective element?

Here, TM begins to look suspicious. As far as the physiological changes detailed are concerned, TM is not unique among relaxation therapies. Other 'self-regulation' strategies such as biofeedback or progressive muscular relaxation are almost certainly as effective. Medically speaking, there is nothing special about TM. Dr Herbert Benson, an Associate Professor at Harvard Medical School, who did much of the early medical research into TM now proposes a simple method (relaxing and silently repeating the word 'one') which gives the same results, can be learned in a minute without a fee, and without TM initiation. There is no proof that sitting back on the sofa with a good book or gentle gardening would not have the same benefits in relaxation! In other words, it is the methodology which works and not the principle.

4. What are the assumptions of the world view behind the therapy?

Maharishi Mahesh Yogi was born around 1918 in Central India, in the Kshatriya (warrior) caste. Little is known of his early life but in 1940 he took a Bachelor's degree in physics at Allahabad University. Until 1953 he sought spiritual enlightenment from his guru, Swami Brahmenanda Saraswati ('Guru Dev' - divine teacher - for short) and from him learned the essence of the yoga techniques he later simplified and offered to the world as TM. When Guru Dev died, the monk Mahesh spent 2 years in caves in the Himalayas meditating and communing with 'Ultimate Reality', before descending from the snowy peaks as a self-proclaimed 'master' with the title 'Maharishi' (Great Sage) 'Mahesh' (family name) 'Yogi' (one who has achieved union with God).

There were plenty of Spiritual Masters in India so the Maharishi shrewdly came West where people are, to quote him, 'in the habit of accepting things quickly'. It was California in the mid-60's and the The Beatles which brought him to prominence in the West.

TM is a deceptive manifestation of Hindu religion. Space does not permit full details. ... For example, before being taught how to practice TM, the initiate brings offerings of a clean white handkerchief, flowers and fruit; removes his or her shoes; and is invited to bow down to a statue or photograph of Guru Dev. He or she is then present while their teacher (and each Teacher of TM is personally inducted by the Maharishi) intones worshipfully a Sanskrit hymn of praise which translated into English, as it never is in the ceremony, reads:

'Guru in the glory of Brahma, Guru in the glory of Vishnu. Guru in the glory of the personified transcendental fulness of Brahman, to Him, to Shri Guru Dev adorned with glory, I bow down'.

Thus there is worship of the traditional Hindu gods, and it is important to realise that the TM Teacher would regard Guru Dev and probably the Maharishi as divine.

TM always denies publicly that it is either a philosophy or a religion, and of Christianity the Maharishi says simply that a Christian practising TM will be a better Christian. However, private comments and the testimonies of those who have abandoned TM, make it clear that it is a religion, and courts in the USA and Medical Ethical Committees in Denmark have ruled that it is a religion and not a medical therapy.

Like a chameleon TM changes its colours to suit the prevailing philosophical climate. Thus it has been sold as a political movement for world peace; as a source of personal or corporate calm and its practice is thus required of its employees by some companies; or, health being the present obsession in the West, as an 'alternative medicine'.

5. Does the therapy involve the occult, that is, practices specifically forbidden in Scripture?

Our God said (Exodus 20 v 1 ff): *'I am the Lord thy God... Thou shall have no other gods before me. Thou shall not make unto thee any graven image... Thou shalt not bow down thyself to them, nor serve them...'* The above makes it clear that the practice of TM requires us to break these commandments.

It is quite possible that as the mind is emptied and the mantra (a secret word of Sanskrit scripture) repeated - itself an act of worship to Hindu deities - that spiritual forces of the Devil come in. The author has read testimonies of people who suffered demonic oppression as a result of TM.

6. Has the therapy stood the test of time?

TM is new, but its meditative and religious or philosophical background has been around for thousands of years. This does not give it credibility. Satan has been busy a long time.

Conclusion

TM produces physiological benefits but these are consequent on the relaxation, and other non-religious relaxation practices will produce equal medical benefits. TM is a religion incompatible with Christianity and it requires us to disobey our Lord and to open our lives to the spiritual forces of evil. Surely Christians must reject it absolutely. ★

Unless we keep our focus on Jesus, our hearts in the word of God as we read it in the Bible, and a balanced view of the Scriptures, Christians can be made to forget that Satan can masquerade as an angel of light. His plan will work for each one of us if we give him a chance. Satan is very subtle. He can begin with any truth. 'Focus on Jesus', he might even say!

I had to learn that Jesus was not just another Mantra. The month immediately prior to my conversion and immediately following the death of my fellow 'searcher', was spent in more searching. But now my search took me to look at the dangers of the occult healing methods I had been involved with. During that month, and prompted by a notice in the magazine of my local Anglican church, I attended a weekend retreat for **contemplative prayer.** This can be an ordinary part of the Christian way of prayer, but I didn't know Jesus, and the repetitive words and thoughts that were the basis of the time spent in the Retreat Chapel can, for me, only have been mantras. However what of the dangers generally with this kind of meditation? Mental passivity provides an open door for the enemy; free-will can diminish with the repetitiveness of whatever is said.

Autosuggestion is another therapy that doesn't need the participating help of another. **Couéism** involved the repetition of the words, 'Every day and in every way, I'm getting better and better.' **Visualisation therapy** is a variety of autosuggestion commonly found today, and used with cancer patients. They are asked to relax, focus on breathing, and to visualise or imagine the cancer under attack until it eventually disappears. Such

★ *Transcendental Meditation - Who Goes Where?* by Dr Andrew Fergusson (Pacemaker, Nurses Christian Fellowship, April 1987)

imagination is the counterfeit of God's faith. From meditation and autosuggestion are developed other therapies. One is a method of **mind control** where there is an emphasis on expanding intuition and extra-sensory perception (ESP). It seems to a be sort of dynamic meditation. It is a counterfiet of listening to God's direction; also ESP is very dangerous - a power to be renounced and repented of by Christians if they find that they have it. Wherever and however the occult is involved, Satan is automatically given the right of access.

From America, Medical Doctor Jane D Gumprecht tells us★ that the latest weapon for mind control in the schools starting in the first grade is 'Q.R.', which means **Quieting Reflex.** The idea is to treat stress and the children are subjected to early states of self-hypnosis. The children are told that stress occurs 'when parents get into the picture' and it is preferable that they go for advice to the 'wise men' who live inside their bodies rather than to parents or to God. Then, still in line with this occult concept of the spirit guide, really a demon but in this case seen as the 'wise men', the children are called upon to breathe slowly through imaginary holes in their feet.

Breathing is significant as an aid to meditation. Meditation techniques involve a focus of attention. The purpose is to come into a state of **passivity,** the basic teaching of Hinduism and Buddhism from which these New Age techniques spring. The centre of attention can be the breathing, a lighted candle, a mandala (which is a geometric design), burning coals in a fire or anything else that's found suitable. The passivity is achieved through blanking the mind by making any situation or object the **centre** of our attention; this gives us the new term, better known in America, to describe meditation.

★ *Holistic Health* (Ransom Press)

It is **centering.** Quieting Reflex is designed to relieve stress, and of course the driving force in the promotion of centering techniques is the idea of relieving stress. As Dr Gumprecht tells us in her medical and biblical critique of the Holistic Health deception, 'stress and burnout' are words that have entered the popular vernacular very quickly. She has found that the holistic health movement is riding on the crest of a wave by using stress as a major vehicle for enticing the uninformed Christian into their treatment regimen. The list can be longer but Dr Gumprecht specifically identifies hypnosis, deep breathing techniques, visualisation, yoga, TM, reflexology, rolfing and energy transference through therapeutic touch, 'laying on of hands', deep massage and guided imagery. These, she says, are used to relieve stress.

Dr Gumprecht explodes the idea of the classic medical condition of the stomach ulcer which has been used to convince the public that the mind and emotions cause physical, organic changes in the body. With a good understanding of Satan's strategy through Hindu beliefs in the New Age, she writes that breaking down the barriers between mind and body (the body/mind concept) is 'crucial' to Satan's strategy for mind control. The concept is that of melding the human mind with Divine mind. 'Divine mind is the god of the New Age... an impersonal force and not the personal Jehovah God revealed in the Bible.'★ Body/mind is the Eastern-Hindu concept of the psycho-soma and the doctor tells us: 'That mind causes illness is foundational to holistic medicine, but the medical establishment doesn't agree. There are no scientific studies that give credence to the concept of the mind causing disease, only that emotions can influence symptomatology or the way a person

★ *Holistic Health* (Ransom Press)

feels.'★ One of the meditation, centering, stress-relieving techniques where the method is akin to the calling forth of 'wise men' in the quieting reflex therapy for children referred to above is guided imagery.

The use of **guided imagery** involves extending the meditative state to create a specific mental picture for diagnosis and healing. Carl Simonton, MD is an advocate of this mental imagery technique. In his book *Getting Well Again* ★★ he encourages patients to locate an 'inner guide'. We are to ask the guide's name, then ask it for help with our problems! It is true that we have natural healing mechanisms within us, but we are headed for danger when we start to see the subconscious as an infallible fountain of wisdom, or psychology (as the word is used today) as anything more than the science of the human soul and mind without God.

Chromotherapy is based upon the idea that every colour has a vibration rate different from that of any other colour. It is thousands of years old and there is a school of 'healers' using colour and music for healing.

Biofeedback describes the measurement of body changes - the sort we are not normally aware of - by using equipment. In the doctor's hands this can be quite legitimate, and the EEG machine for measuring brain-wave patterns is an example. The new application is in alternative medicine. Small versions of the EEG machine are available relatively inexpensively with a display panel so that the performance can be clearly seen. Meditators are encouraged to reach the so-called higher states of consciousness and trance previously only

★ *Holistic Health* (Ransom Press)

★★ *Getting Well Again* by O Carl Simonton MD, Stephanie Matthews-Simonton and James L Creighton (Bantam Books, 666 Fifth Avenue, New York, NY 10103)

experienced by eastern gurus and holy men.

I used to sit, both in sessions with my guru and in my own office, wired up to the biofeedback equipment. Dave Hunt is an internationally recognised cult expert; his extensive research has taken him to over forty countries, and the following is how he sees the enormous significance of biofeedback in the context of what he calls New Age occult technology:

> Western technology has invented, designed manufactured, and marketed, commercial devices for automatically producing the so-called 'higher' states of consciousness that open the door to occult experiences and psychic powers. What used to take a powerful dose of LSD or months of yoga, meditation and vegetarianism can now be accomplished in a few minutes through new devices that are multiplying at an alarming rate. Biofeedback was one of the first such mechanisms. That those who developed it realised what they were doing is indicated by the fact that biofeedback is called 'electronic yoga.' The Menninger Clinic of Topeka, Kansas, has a promotional film titled 'Biofeedback, the Yoga of the West.' In other words biofeedback puts you in the same state of consciousness and develops the same control over involuntary bodily functions - and the same occult experiences and psychic powers - that have been the stock in trade of great Yogis since the Garden of Eden. ★

With science on the side of the meditators, it is no longer necessary to spend half a lifetime in a yoga position

★ Taken from *Peace, Prosperity & The Coming Holocaust*, copyright © 1983. Harvest House Publishers, 1075 Arrowsmith, Eugene. OR 97405, USA Used by permission.

staring into a fire in a Himalayan cave. The path to enlightenment, by way of the full awareness of all other Hindu beliefs, which we look at in Chapter Eleven, is much speeded up in these days.

I believe it will now be becoming clear that the traditional ways of Hinduism permeate alternative medicine. It will have its relevance in medical science too, but that is an area for separate study. However one therapy ought to be mentioned here, and that is the **placebo.** Studies show that large numbers of patients get better when given tablets known by the doctors to be useless, and these are called placebos. Is such faith well placed? Believe in it and it will work! Here we have the basis for a whole range of psychological pick-me-ups. It is true that many of these therapies, like the simple placebo, are not dangerous like TM or hypnosis. However, Christians will see many of them as poor attempts by man to organise God out of health care, and it is doubtful if much is achieved. Another psychological therapy in the field of alternative medicine is **auto-genics.** This involves easy mental exercises to switch 'from the stress system to the rest, relaxation and re-creation system.'

The therapies so far identified are solutions centred on 'self'. The 'self-realisation' of the higher state of consciousness of the east is similar to psychology's faith in such self-help techniques as go under the heading of **psychotherapy.** In his book, *Psychology as Religion,* ★ Paul Vitz, a Professor of Psychology, clearly presents psychology as the 'cult of self-worship'. Freud gave us **psychoanalysis.** This is a way of examining the soul! It involves a probing deep into the subconcious, thought life, imagination and unclean sexual dreams. The idea is one of discovery through an unhealthy method of

★ *Psychology as Religion - the Cult of Self Worship* by Paul C Vitz (Lion) - 1977.

looking inwards, and the search is for the cause of psychic and moral disorders. By ignoring or denying the relationship of sin and sickness, psychoanalysis hinders or destroys the healthy and biblical faith in Jesus. The mistake is the belief that wrongs can be put right if only we can discover ourselves. After Freud, Jung devoted himself to 'self-understanding' and 'self-realisation.' As with all psychology, reckoning man's behaviour apart from a knowledge of Jesus, these famous men have substantially failed in their task.

We find psychoanalysis at the root of techniques such as **dream therapy.** This is a group therapy where, one by one, the other members provide a commentary on the dream and where the dreamer can decide which, if any, fits!

In another psychological category, perhaps somewhat more acceptable, are the behavioural therapies such as **aversion therapy** where, for example, a drug given to an alcoholic is designed to make him sick if he drinks alcohol. However when we come to therapies grounded in humanistic psychology we find a minefield of danger. **Metamorphic technique** is based upon reflexology and works on points of the feet and **elsewhere** that are supposed to relate to the nine-month cycle of prenatal growth. Another is **primal therapy,** or Rebirthing (discussed in Chapter Five). This seeks to discover problems arising from the time in the womb, using hypnotic age regression, psychedelics like LSD, simulation of the birth experience or breathing. **Inner healing,** as practised by Christians, has stumbled into this Satanic realm. In some forms of it self-discovery exercises and occult-related therapies more akin to the human potential movement are practised, and the subject of wrong Christian involvement with inner healing is explored further in Chapter Fifteen.

Rogerian therapy is said to be a path to 'self-actualisation' and trust in one's own inner growth.

Encounter therapy, also to be avoided, is a development from this, emphasising physical expression. **Gestalt** is another with the aim of 'self-discovery' and 'self-liberation'. To throw off inhibitions there is **psychodrama** where problems can be acted out, and another therapy designed to uncover what we really feel is **transactional analysis.** Another is **co-counselling,** a recognised therapy where people help one another. **Clinical theology** is an approach promoted by the Clinical Theology Association. This exists for training people in counselling, and for the deepening of Christain life and growth towards personal maturity and stability. There is also provision in the Association's 'objects' for research 'into the integration of psychology and psychotherapy with the Christian faith.' Whilst the Association is an ecumencial Christian foundation, they do seem to believe not only in the respect for *people* with different beliefs (entirely right and proper according to Scripture), but also for personal convictions and religious heritages different from ours, as reflecting the freedom God gives to men and women. They regard the joint research of helper and person seeking help, for firmer and deeper resources of meaning *within the counselee's own beliefs,* to be one of the important functions of counselling.

The Oxford Dictionary description of 'occult' is about the most useful I have seen: 'Kept secret, esoteric; recondite, mysterious, beyond the range of ordinary knowledge; involving the supernatural, mystical, magical.' As ever, the line is difficult to draw, but on any view it can be no part of my position to assert that the tools provided by transactional analysis and clinical theology qualify for that description. They are included because they involve therapies, as it were 'alternative' to what the doctor or psychiatrist might otherwise be called upon to provide. They are included also for the reason that Christians will sometimes turn from the 'drug' remedies, not only to the so-called 'natural' remedies, but also to the 'psychological'.

Clinical theology, founded by a psychiatrist in 1960 has always had good standing among church people. Transactional analysis was also originated by a psychiatrist, and in 1980 the Church of Scotland published *A Tool for Christians* to teach its use. The book described the subject in this way:

> Transactional Analysis is not 'Christian'. It is a secular theory of observable human behaviour and personality. It happens to be a theory which can be used within a Christian framework for it highlights much of what the New Testament teaches about human relationships. It is not a theology - it does not teach about God; but many of its insights can be of value to the modern Christian working out how to love his neighbour as himself.

Some will be helped to grow in their Christian life through transactional analysis, clinical theology, and other therapies that have their roots in psychology. However, we have to take care that we go God's way and not man's way. Psychology shifts us man's way; the Bible will take us God's way.

East meets West in the final categorisation of psychological therapy, **transpersonal psychology.** This is the psychology of 'transcendent experience', and therapists practising **psychosynthesis** attempt to harmonise the creation of a so-called healthy western-style personality with the Eastern emphasis on higher levels of consciousness.

Emile Krémer★ tells us that **group dynamics** (or 'group therapy' or 'sensitivity training') has been

---

★ *Eyes Opened to Satan's Subtlety* by Emile Krémer (MOVE Press 1969).

rapidly spreading in the west for many years, not only in social, economic, scientific and political training centres but also in churches and Christian circles. There are groups under various names such as **group psycho-therapy** and **interpersonal relationship,** as well as the encounter groups and transactional analysis mentioned previously. It is actually a form of 'brainwashing' and it is in some contrast to the Christian community where unity is through Jesus Christ and the focus of all upon him.

Born out of the ideas to be found in psychology, we hear much about **positive thinking** in relation to health. The Christian has a positive attitude, not because of his belief in the power there certainly is in positive thinking, but because he is trusting God. On the other hand the thinking of the human potential movement, advanced by many, can be identified in the Association of Humanistic Psychology. This is a world-wide network formed in 1962 for the development of the so-called human sciences in ways that recognise our human 'qualities' and which work towards fulfilling our 'innate' capacities. It explores human potential on the basis that it is infinite.

Many Christian leaders today are bringing a message that has its roots in humanistic psychology and eastern religion. For Christians there can be a subtle and dangerous path which is a departure from trusting God. It leads back through **positive confession,** a Christian based movement looked at in Chapter Fifteen, and on to the **positive mental attitude** ideas and positive thinking identified here.

With *God* all things are possible. The *human potential movement* embracing many of the therapies in this chapter, takes the view, either that we don't *need* God, or that we *are* God. They believe that with *man* all things are possible. Indeed man is very powerful. Irrespective of what we believe in, we can make things happen by believing. The Christian way is quite different.

The *Daily Telegraph* reported (26 November 1984) that the teaching of fire-walking was coming to Britain: 'The other evening near Los Angeles she led a group of more than forty barefoot participants as they strode through an 8' pit of burning embers with a temperature of 1,300 degrees Fahrenheit. None suffered more than the odd blister.' It is Satanic. Some will be badly burned, but the price to be paid in the spiritual realm is even worse. Such is the human potential movement. While the world wonders, thank God for the discernment He gives to Christians on these things. Evidently there has been little 'scientific research' on this fire-walking! The article concludes: '... one theory holds that the feet have a cushion of surface moisture which vaporises to form an insulating cushion of steam for the very short duration of the walk'.

Like the voice of a departed relative or the ectoplasmic manifestation of his or her body, this human potential is in one sense real enough. But the Christian should be able to recognise it as a counterfeit.

We have no worthwhile potential without Jesus. Indeed without Him we have a potential for Satan. Such is the guise of the human potential movement. The answer is in knowing both the character of God and the character of Satan.

7
Paranormal therapies

This is a description given by modern secular writers to the group of 'healing' therapies they can't understand in terms of pseudo-science, energy charts, astrology or whatever. We even see divine healing sometimes lumped in with the rest! The spiritually blind cannot see the difference between the real and the counterfeit.

Every occult method is dangerous and an undue categorisation of Satan's deceptions is undesirable. Also it isn't logical to go to great lengths comparing methods which anyway have their roots with spirits who are intentionally deceptive. However the broad headings of therapies in this part of the book will assist Christian understanding. While secular writers on 'alternative medicine' are separating the paranormal and the psychic from the rest and conceding 'we don't yet fully understand...', discerning Christians are indentifying the spiritual however it is disguised.

It is clear that involvement with some of the paranormal therapies in this particular section brings the patient into contact with practitioners powerfully gripped by Satan.

Spiritualist healing is very dangerous indeed. Healing which is not God's, in the name of Jesus, is Satan's. Such healing is found in Spiritualist churches, in so-called Christian Spiritualist churches, and in some so-called Christian churches where the fellowship either doesn't know Jesus or where it is simply undiscerning. Satan is behind every variation that is to be found. Some call themselves **psychic healers.** Others style themselves as **faith healers.** Then there are **hand healers.** Often the same people engage in **absent healing.** Christians don't have to be present with a patient in order to pray for him; neither do the practitioners of the counterfeits when they engage in absent healing. One healing network spells out a procedure of self-visualisation, starting with the feet and moving on throughout the body. Perhaps hundreds or even thousands in this particular network are doing this at the same time each week. Then fifteen minutes later they all move into the 'Healing time' when they visualise all the others in the network sending them 'light' and 'love'! They bring into their imagination anyone they know who needs help and healing. They visualise them as filled with selfless love and light. The idea is that the more people there are in the group the better. They emphasise it has nothing to do with religion but that human beings are helping each other with love. According to the network, some call it 'spirit' and some call it 'synergy'. Whatever they call it, the source of any apparent healing is quite clear. They are opening themselves up to the activities of demons.

Another area where the hands are involved is **magnetic healing.** It has nothing to do with magnets. Yet one practitioner I have seen *does* use magnets for healing! There is a British Bio-magentic Association which runs Seminars on **healing with magnets.**

Some healers go into trance or altered state of consciousness. They make contact with what they call 'spirit guides'. They either believe they are possessed by them or simply that the guides take over their movements and leave their minds clear. The 'Healer' may get verbal instructions from demons by clairaudience, or he may see the problem and its explanation by a sort of x-ray experience — clairvoyance. Given the diagnosis, the healing may be brought about by hand passes, or however the 'spirit' leads. Healers vary in their beliefs and techniques. Indeed the variety is a parallel counterfeit to the multiple methods of healing that Jesus used.

Some healers in the spirit of the New Age movement, are interested in the so-called scientific explanation of the healing and they don't need to identify with any religious notion of a spirit guide.

Whatever the variations in description, we can indentify this sort of healing as psychic, coming from the 'psyche' (Gk. soul). The soul is made up of mind, will and emotions, and psychic healing comes from the mind rather than the spirit. The spirit of the Christian is occupied by the Holy Spirit, that same Holy Spirit that indwells all born again believers. Divine healing involves the Holy Spirit.

The use of the term 'spiritual healing' or 'spiritualist healing' may imply that the spirit of the healer is taken over by, in this case, a demonic spirit. However 'faith healers', 'spiritual healers' and all the rest of them, usually using the laying on of hands, have often little to distinguish them. Clearly there can be those powerfully possessed by demons.

Also in so-called charismatic fellowships of Bible-believing Christians, some put the wrong emphasis on the 'psyche', where the Holy Spirit is absent and where there is no discernment as to the source of the power. If our faith is centred on Jesus, His word and His will in each situation, if the occult is not involved, and if the healing is in the name of Jesus by people who know Jesus, then we should have nothing to fear.

What of **psychic surgery?** Many wonder if it is an illusion when the psychic surgeon in Mexico uses a dirty knife to open up a patient's body, and when the wound immediately is sealed at the close of an operation during which extraordinary foreign bodies have been removed; or when, in the Philippines, the patient's body is opened up, in the view of qualified medical investigators, with no cutting instruments used. It is *not* an illusion. It is *not* nonsense. In these days too, even western man is seeking out the 'genuine' **witchdoctor** or **shaman.** In Satan's plan the witch still curses and the witchdoctor, as the name implies, still 'heals'.

Our own pagan practices, like the **charming of warts** and **copper bracelets** for rheumatism, must also be renounced by Christians. Another self-healing method is with crystals, and no doubt it can be fairly described as **crystal therapy!** One practitioner teaches that we should sit quietly, then focus on places of pain and tension in the body. Next we place a crystal we 'feel attracted to', either directly on the place that needs it, or in the left hand, 'allowing the left hand to place the crystal "intuitively" on the part of the body that needs it.' He continues, 'At the "Crystal Explorer Groups" currently held twice weekly... one can go far deeper, with loving support, into crystal energies.' We can put our faith in anything in order to get results! **Pattern therapy** assumes patterns or shapes can help cure disease. The same goes for **pyramid healing.** Pyramid power was important to the pharaohs, and occultists use it today.

Ayurveda from India is perhaps the oldest medical discipline. It is rooted in the occult. The Greeks picked up aspects of it, and much of our own medicine came from Greece. As for India, ayurveda is still responsible for most health care in that country today. It is endorsed by the World Health Organisation, and ayurvedic medicine now has its own association in Britain.

Therapeutic touch, found in a whole range of practitioners in these days, is a good example of the ancient energy concept of 'prana' dressed for acceptibility today. It is even taught to some nurses. It is listed here in the 'paranormal' section since arm waving around the body, without any touch at all, is quite common in this therapy. It is a therapy most readily grasped by those who have looked in on yoga or the martial arts. **Applied kinesiology** is optional teaching in some chiropractic training schools and 'touch for health', referred to in Chapter Five is a well known therapy under this heading. Once again touch may not be touch at all. Directing to the so-called aura or etheric body, some will simply make a hand pass and wave it close to the skin.

Derived from applied kinesiology is **behavioural kinesiology.** This attempts to demonstrate with a so-called 'arm strength test', how food, clothes, art and various other factors cause fluctuations in 'life energy'. Names! Names! In Satan's plan, the more the better. 'Bio' prefixes much in science and mecicine, and so it is also in occult medicine! One treatment is **biokinesiology;** a Christian G P described to me the procedure of one practitioner she knows: The idea was to identify dietary substances which would be harmful to the patient. Small amounts of the substance under test were in turn placed upon the subject's tongue whilst the practitioner attempted to lower the subject's arm as it was held extended first above the head, then about waist level, and then lower. Apparently it was quite easy for the subject to resist these attempts to move his arm, except when any dietary substance 'harmful' to him was placed upon his tongue when he seemed powerless to resist the force applied by the practitioner. Then a similar procedure was repeated, but this time instead of the substance being placed on the tongue they remained in their unopened bottle and the bottle was placed on the skin of the abdomen. This had the same apparent effect on muscle power, and the harmful substances thus identified were the same in both instances - fish, tea, sugar and monosodium glutamate.

Neurologists properly tell us that muscle power in the same individual will vary and depend most of all on his *will* to resist. It is also true that we once again have the deception of the common denominator found in so much of the paranormal — 'energy'. The word biokinesiology is derived from 'kinetic' (energy; Gk. 'kinetikos') but it is a counterfeit; for it to be otherwise, as one Christian writer★ on this has put it, it seems every textbook on physiology would have to be rewritten.

The spiritual healing to be found in **Christian Science** is neither Christian nor scientific and has to be avoided. Satan will sometimes heal through Christian Science. Satan and sin can cause sickness and Satan can certainly take away the symptoms to accommodate the cultists and get a better hold on the gullible. Satan always has a high price — mental breakdown, suicide, oppression, etc.

Finally I introduce to you **past lives therapy!** Patients are asked by the therapist to recreate scenes in past lives for the supposed purpose of understanding the present problems. It is a Satanic deception, and of course the evil one can also provide the scenes.

These paranormal therapies have, in one subtle way and another, introduced through alternative medicine numerous aspects of Hindu doctrine set up by Satan to deceive us. Yet to some of us, past lives therapy isn't really that subtle! Satan would like us to forget any idea of hell as he advertises a 'next life' after this one. The idea is prompted just as well by the concept of a 'past life!' The view that we are indeed in the last of the last days is supported by the way that these more blatant lies are received by the intelligent. More and more are being deceived, Christian and non-Christian alike.

★ *The Holistic Healers* by Paul C Reisser, MD, Teri K Reisser and John Weldon. Inter Varsity Press, Downers Grove, Illinois 60515, USA (1983).

8
Paranormal diagnosis

In the field of **psychic diagnosis** the foremost figure was Edgar Cayce. His trance states provided very accurate diagnosis. Psychics can be very accurate today and they are more and more consulted by doctors who are themselves deceived. To be a receiver of treatment following this diagnosis is not to be distant from Satan's influence. Any sort of involvement with the methods of Satan, either directly or indirectly, intentionally or not, is very dangerous.

Radiesthesia is a pseudo-scientific term meaning the perception of radiations which are said to emanate from everything that exists. Some are into this invisible world without needing a pendulum or other device. They see by **clairvoyance** or hear by **clairaudience.** Deceiving spirits answer the enquirer, and those already opened up through superstitions, charming or other occult practices are sometimes able to progress quickly in these counterfeit gifts. Often these gifts come down a family line. The Bible says that sins are visited on future generations, and children who have received **inherited powers** will retain them until they are renounced and until they repent. Typically a **pendulum** is used in diagnosis. For example, when I moved my pendulum down the spinal cord of one of my subjects, a swing in the reverse direction would be expected where the problem was located and the energy out of balance. Once again results are ascribed to energy or radiations without any attempt to describe their nature or prove their existence. The same explanations are given for water divining (or 'water witching' or 'water dowsing'); but when asked to explain the success at dowsing from maps, practitioners are forced to abandon this reasoning.

For the mechanically minded, radiesthesia can become **radionics.** Human hair or some other body element is shown to the machine! A modern-day encyclopaedia of 'natural health and healing' describes the apparatus as using the thought of the skilled operator as a probe in determining the basic causes of ill-health. What next! Some of these modern-day diviners will use **psychometry.** This involves giving a body sample, again hair or anything else, to a perhaps absent practitioner.

Kirlian photography can show the Kirlian practitioner a photographed aura of his patient. This is the halo effect said to represent the etheric body and is akin to the aura that many psychics can see around the human body. They really do see auras. Like poltergeists, they are manifestations to further the purpose of keeping man away from God. The Kirlian photograph is made of the fingers, and the interpretation is based upon the patterns and colours in the photograph. It is a modern version of **palmistry,** itself occult, and still used for diagnosis. **Mediumistic iridology** (or 'eye diagnosis'), using the eye rather like a crystal ball, is another source for diagnosis used by therapists with half-baked scientific ideas and spiritually deceived.

Astrologic medicine is a form of divination based on the belief that signs - in this case of the sun, moon and planets in the lines of the zodiac - correspond to lines of physical, mental, emotional and spiritual well-being. Astronomy is a science; astrology is occult. **Biorhythms** is another deception increasingly looked at by alternative practitioners. It holds that there are three body cycles (physical - 23 days; emotional - 28 days; intellectual - 33 days) running from birth to death. The idea is to know when to avoid stressful occasions and potential illness. Its charts, like those in astrology, are for the curious and seem to have no basis in science.

Whilst some psychics do not need a pendulum or any sort of equipment at all, the world takes time examining the equipment! Doctors take time examining the results! There even exists the Psionic Medicine Society. An additional professional qualification is offered to doctors and dentists by the Institute of Psionic Medicine. This extension of the medical profession seems to offer an integrated system linking orthodox medicine, homoeopathy and radiesthesia. It is all relatively new. The Society was formed in 1968. Except on the basis of 'It doesn't work!', like so much in alternative medicine, it seems to go substantially unchallenged by the medical profession.

9

Homoeopathy

This is a branch of medicine based on herbs and minerals. It uses highly diluted solutions said to become more powerful the greater the dilution. The power of the solution is further believed to depend upon shaking to release the drug's energy. There appears to be no accepted scientific base for Hahnemann's application of these ideas. (Hahnemann was the founder of homoeopathy).

Homoeopathy arrived in Britain around 1840. It was introduced by a Dr Quin who is said to have had influential friends. Eventually the London Homoeopathic Hospital acquired its 'Royal' status. Sir John Weir was appointed personal physician and served four monarchs for forty-eight years until 1971. There is still a homoeopathic physician serving the Royal Family today and most homoeopathic doctors are believed to acknowledge that the Royal Family has helped to keep homoeopathy alive in Britain.

Homoeopathy is thus established in the ranks of a medical profession dominated by the question: 'does it work?' While answers are being sought to that question (both in this and other areas of counterfeit healing) the spiritual aspect continues to be missed. Satan smiles!

Hahnemann was deceived. After 150 years man still hasn't found his scientific answer, and the deception has continued. Satan has blinded to the truth of it. It thrives in India! In Britain it survives! By and large doctors don't like what they see as an absence of science; but it is much worse than that!

Before any so-called intellectual approach I believe God spoke to me according to the testimony I relate below. But first a cautionary word about testimonies.

A cautionary word about testimonies

Whilst writing this book and endeavouring to take a great deal of care with scriptures, checking and rechecking manuscripts with those who know their Bibles well, I do not escape the fact that I am not a Bible scholar myself. The danger of that position can be the tendency to rely excessively on what is commonly called testimony and what might more helpfully be described as experiences. I have known that trap; apart from an understanding of the Word of God, it is all too easy to major on testimony — on experiences.★ It is better to bring the focus, seen in this chapter, on what homoeopathy is and what the Bible says. God can speak to each one of us through very different circumstances and as can be seen in the testimonies that follow.

Personal testimony

Attending a Christian conference, a friend pointed out a Christian doctor to me. 'He's a homoeopathic doctor', I was told much to my surprise. It seemed to be a nudge from God for, just an hour before, in another place, I had also been taken aback.

En route to the conference I had thumbed through a

★ *Understanding Deception.*

new Christian exposé of psychic healing.★ Homoeopathy had been lumped in with what were described as 'fascinatingly named healing alternatives'. There they were — iridology, astrologic medicine, colour therapy, sound therapy, radionics, kinesiology, orgonomy, biofeedback, 'past lives' therapy, zone therapy, rolfing, polarity therapy, Kirlian photography, to name just a few. I had been involved with some of them; they were occult. I had given some of them a miss but I knew they were occult. Some I sensed were occult, but I didn't know for sure. Homoeopathy, although not among those the author singled out as positively occult (I later learned he hadn't yet researched it fully), had seemed to be the odd man out.

I had passed the Bristol Homoeopathic Hospital every day on my way to the university. Very respectable it had all seemed. So I was surprised by the book, and just an hour later — after reading it and now sitting in the conference hall — it seemed God was directing me to a Christian homoeopathic doctor.

My friend gave me the doctor's name and address. Was God telling me that homoeopathy was not of Him? Or was he telling me to seek the advice of the Christian homoeopathic doctor? I knew that people involved in the occult could not be good witnesses, Christian or not. It was no time to consult the doctor! I waited upon the Lord.

Several months passed. Although living a good distance from the doctor, circumstances brought us together and we came to know one another on a continuing basis. I shared my concern about homoeopathy with him. 'Homoeopathy is certainly of God', he assured me. It was time to wait upon the Lord once again.

★ *Psychic Healing - an exposé of an occult phenomenon by* John Weldon and Zola Levitt (Moody Press, Chicago, USA) 1982.

More months passed. I was seated outside a café in Brussels. A young Dutch Christian, whom I didn't know, came and sat beside me. Somehow the subject of homoeopathy — not in my thoughts for a long time — came into the conversation. He gave me what at the time seemed the most extraordinary reason why he went to medical school. He wanted to get to the bottom of a whole area of occult medicine that included Paracelsus and homoeopathy. To me the explanations were very technical, but it seemed clear he had succeeded. He had done the research. Although I didn't understand fully, I was quite clear in my spirit, as he was in his, that homoeopathy was indeed occult.

Two days later, and back at home, an evangelist moved in with us for a few days. In the days immediately before (while I was learning from my new Dutch friend) she had been staying with the homoeopathic doctor who, by this time, had become a good friend of mine. The visitor to our home brought good news. She had discerned the spirit of homoeopathy. More than that, the Lord had spoken at the same time to my good friend. She told me he had renounced homoeopathy. He had destroyed the equipment and his homoeopathic medicines.

Homoeopathy (and not just the occult practices that sometimes accompany it) is from deceiving spirits.

My book, *Beware Alternative Medicine,* published in 1983, was, as far as I am aware the first Christian book in the English language which stated unequivocally that homoeopathy was from deceiving spirits and was occult. I relate that only to evidence the grip that Satan has had, and the measure of the deception there has been since homoeopathy arrived in Britain around 1840. This is all the more remarkable given the extraordinary things witnessed in homoeopathy by the well-qualified and highly educated people who head up the homoeopathy fraternity in Britain. ★

Testimony of the doctor mentioned above

The following is an extract from the testimony of the doctor, a Consultant Ophthalmologist, mentioned above. It originally appeared in the forewords of the previous editions of this book.

> "Roy Livesey, in this unique book, is opening our eyes to Satan's deceptions. They look good and give results but come from the wrong source and the wrong power. As the doctor in the testimony Roy writes on homoeopathy, I can say that, since renouncing homoeopathy as occult, I have found my relationship with Jesus much more real and effective. I am seeing Him heal as I pray against sickness in His name, something I had come to accept would never be my experience.
> Homoeopathy, though producing results, had robbed me of faith in the hightest source of healing: Jesus Christ the Son of God.
> Roy has been very courageous in presenting the truth. Although this truth may offend some, I trust that for many it will be the truth that sets them free."

The testimonies of others

Since the date of my own testimony, I have received testimonies from others. The following was written by another Christian doctor:

★ *Understanding Deception.*

In the experience of many patients, and overtly in various TV programmes on homoeopathy, the pendulum is being used; definitely an occult practice. Moreover, in our experience several Spirit-filled patients have not 'benefited' from homoeopathy but have actually had severe and damaging reactions to the treatment and their condition has deteriorated — remarkable considering that physically there is probably only sugar and water in the medication. (Testimonies can be given).

We have also found that involvement with Homoeopathy has been one of the factors in preventing people from moving forward in their relationship with God, into the fullness of the Holy Spirit, and their new inheritance in Christ Jesus (Mark 16:17-18; Rom. 8:14-17).

She concludes by saying that homoeopathy itself (as well as the pendulum) is something for which repentance is necessary. It has to be renounced, like all occult therapies, whenever there has been involvement.

In these days Christians caught up in the apostasy about which the Bible warns are singing the praises of homoeopathy. One Christian practitioner of Homoeopathy who renounced it and gave her testimony in 1987★ thought that as many as seventy-five per cent of Christians in her area were involved with homoeopathy.

This lady's testimony is exceptional because eighteen months previously she had, in her own words "defended the battalions of homoeopathy against Andrew Macaulay of Reachout★★, a Christian ministry to people in the

★ This testimony appears in full in *Understanding Deception* by Roy Livesey (New Wine Press, 1987) pages 141-146.

★★ *Reachout Trust* - News letters published by Reachout, PO Box 43, Twickenham, Middx. TW2 7EG.

cults". That was in the magazine "Christian Woman". When homoeopathy was renounced by her, coverage was given in the newspaper "Christian Herald" and the grip this therapy has could be seen reflected in the subsequent letters published by the paper. One of the letters was written by Dr R T Kendall, Minister of the renowned Westminster Chapel in London:

> "Dear Editor: I write to express my concern over a front page piece which gave considerable prominence to a woman who claims to have given up homoeopathic practice owing to it being occult.
> You must know that one of my predecessors, Dr Martyn Lloyd-Jones, was not only a medical doctor but an ardent believer in homoeopathy. He also was a close friend of Dr Margery Blackie who was the Queen's homoeopathic physician and was once a member of Westminster Chapel.
> I might add also that one of Dr Blackie's successors is in the membership at Westminster Chapel and is widely respected by the Christian community." ★

There are many like Dr Lloyd-Jones who are properly respected by Christians, yet as Watchman Nee once wrote, Christian leaders do need to realise that they *can* be deceived.

In another letter to the same newspaper we read: "If homoeopathy is occult, then George Muller of Bristol was deceived." ★ Another wrote; "I cannot believe hundreds of saints of God have been deceived by Satan." ★ Doug Harris, Director of Reachout put his finger on *how* Christians should address this question, and in his letter he wrote:

★ *Christian Herald* (No 12 1987).

"... If after determining the source and the power of homoeopathy you feel you can still use it, that is between you and the Lord. But don't be ignorant of Satan, who is often disguised as an angel of light." ★

Once again, we *all* need to realise that we *can* be deceived.

As we shall see, Hahnemann's "Organ", a document that is still the focus for homoeopaths today, serves also as a bible for them. To Hahnemann illnesses were merely "spiritual, dynamic disturbances of life." ★★ Hence medicine had to be spiritual and dynamic and this is the key to the philosophy.

The Royal Family and Homoeopathy

In my book "Understanding Deception" I wrote about homoeopathy under the chapter title "Homoeopathy - Flagship of Holistic Deception." This described the status given to homoeopathy and its leading role among alternative therapies. In a book about the psychic involvement of the Prince of Wales and other members of the royal family, "The Prince and the Paranormal", there is a chapter with the title "Homoeopathy: The Royal Key." Is homoeopathy the key to the occult involvements of members of the royal family over the past hundred or so years?

Homoeopathy in the disguise of improved herbalism is being used to lead Christians into deception. The perspective of "The Prince and the Paranormal" is not a

★   *Christian Herald* (No 12 1987).

★★   Section 31 of the *Organ* (6th Edition) - translated from the German.

110

Christian one, yet with a researcher's clarity of view John Dale puts his finger on what may well be a key to the blindness to the truth in the face of demonic deception long evidenced in the Royal Family and now more in the open through the boldness of the Prince of Wales. Introducing the subject of Royal involvement in homoeopathy we read:

> "If there is one unusual enthusiasm for which the Royal Family is known, then that enthusiasm is homoeopathy. It is used regularly by the present generation of Royalty, particulary the Queen. And the royal bloodline reaches right back to the discipline's founder, Samuel Hahnemann.
> What is interesting about homoeopathy is the insight it gives us into the Royal Family's attitude to the paranormal."★

Tracing the royal connection John Dale tells us that the first member of the British Royal Family Queen Adelaide was treated in 1835 when a close colleague of Hahnemann's came to London to see her. The most important British homoeopath was Dr Quin. "Despite powerful support, he was called a quack, challenged on legal grounds and received 44 blackballs - a record - when put up for membership of the Athenaeum Club. But he remained popular where it mattered - with his patients - and flourished. He became a figure in aristocratic circles and was a regular guest at the Prince of Wales's dinner table. Among his patients was Princess Mary Adelaide - niece of Queen Adelaide and great-great-grandmother of Prince Charles. It is from this woman that the interest of today's royals directly

★ *The Prince and The Paranormal - The Psychic Bloodline of the Royal Family* by John Dale (W H Allen, London - 1986).

stems... The present Queen carries a small box of homoeopathic remedies with her on her travels; belladonna for her sinusitis, and arsenic to prevent her sneezing in mid-speech. And more recently Prince Charles has been following closely the experimental use of homoeopathic remedies on pigs and cattle at the Elm Farm Research Centre, near Newbury." ★

Homoeopaths prescribe what they call the 'molecular shadow', something more powerful than the bio-chemical effect, and in John Dale's words:

> "...their remedies rely upon a spiritual 'force', not a material one. In this way, homoeopathy is unquestion-ably paranormal."

I include this quotation, taken from "Homoeopathy: the Royal Key", the chapter setting out the royal involvement in "The Prince and the Paranormal", because the chapter appeared in full and without changes in "Homoeopathy" which is the Journal of the British Homoeopathic Association (BHA). As the BHA has the Queen Mother as patron, I think we can take publication by them as confirmation of the facts of royal involvement as detailed in the book. Whilst not publishing Dale's next following chapter, "Royalty, Homoeopathy and the Occult," in the BHA Journal, enough had been written not only to fill in the detail of royal involvement for over 150 years but to sound warning bells, at least to Christians, about the occult nature of the therapy.

Divine healing is the true healing of the supernatural realm. Divine healing is not through some paranormal spiritual 'force', as suggested by the quotation above but through faith in Jesus.

★ *The Prince and The Paranormal.*

Treating the whole person

Homoeopathy has the aim that it seeks to treat the patient as a whole; an attraction shared with the ayurvedic doctor and a counterfeit of what Jesus died to provide — a so-called 'holistic' medicine rather than authentic wholeness.

It has success with patients because it is presented as a treatment that is both personal and scientific, with a remedy both individual and natural. Patients seem readily to receive it in that way. Faced with the routines and mysteries that are in medical science also, patients are tempted to flit from one doctor to another without finding real help; then they find the homoeopath and the holistic approach. Usually they don't know that what they have found is a counterfeit.

One of the happy consequences since the First Edition of this book has been the growth in awareness of the dangers of homoeopathy. This has been evident from the correspondence and comment here, in the United States and around the world.

Homoeopathy seems to be gaining ground along with most of the other alternative medicines. The so-called advantage of the homoeopathic doctor giving more time to the patient than his orthodox counterpart continues to be an important factor. However, on a less personal note, one firm is offering homoeopathic computers with a repertory of 9,000 symptoms and over 500 classical remedies!

Christians, however, are on their guard! So far as I am aware, the first book published in the English language, dealing with both the scientific evaluation *and* the occult connection, was published in 1984. It is *Homeopathy*★ by H J Bopp MD, of Neuchatel, Switzerland, and he

★   HOMEOPATHY without the 'o' is the American spelling.

encourages the Christian, seeking to walk in the light and in obedience to his Lord, not to allow himself to be seduced by every brand of the 'in' philosophy and practice, especially when it comes to finding help for his body, the temple of the Holy Spirit (1 Cor. 6:19). That is why it is so important to look at the history, doctrinal origins and basis of homoeopathy.

History

In the classic study of magic and religion which first appeared in 1890, Sir James Frazer, FRS, FBA, analysed the principles of thought on which magic is based and concluded that broadly there were two principles. His 971-page volume★ identifies the principle that things which have once been in contact with each other continue to act on each other at a distance after the physical contact has been severed. The second principle is that like produces like, or that an effect resembles its cause. Frazer calls this homoeopathic or imitative magic, and shows how the real thing can be affected by the imitation. He cites what is perhaps the best-known example of this principle: 'Perhaps the most familiar application of the principle that like produces like is the attempt which has been made by many peoples in many ages to injure or destroy an enemy by injuring or destroying an image of him, in the belief that, just as the image suffers, so does the man, and that when it perishes he must die.' In other words it is a principle of homoeopathic magic that you don't deal with the real, whether the enemy or the disease, but introduce something like it.

Disease is our enemy today, and it was Paracelsus in

★ *The Golden Bough: A study in Magic & Religion* by J G Frazer (MacMillian & Co) - 1960.

the sixteenth century who was the first to bring mystical research into the area of medicine. He sought to overthrow the classical idea of treating with opposites, with us since Galen (138-201 AD) and still the basis of orthodox medicine today. The ideas of Paracelsus were picked up 300 years later by Samuel Hahnemann, the founder of homoeopathy such as it is practised today. According to the French encyclopedia *Larousse du XXe siècle* (1930) he was believed to have received it through the 'revelation of heavenly powers.'

Doctrine in homoeopathy

In 1810 Hahnemann published what is still today the basis for all homoeopathic treatment: *Organ of the Art of Healing*. This marked a total break with classical and orthodox medicine. The Montreux International Congress on Homoeopathy in 1960 celebrated the 150th anniversary of the *Organ*, and the nostalgia of the event provided the opportunity to see the up-to-date doctrinal views of homoeopathic doctors put on the record. The organiser summed up the *Organ* with these words: 'The *Organ* is for the homoeopath what the Bible is for the Christian. Homoeopathy must consider the *Organ* as the foundation and basis of its therapy.' Dr Bopp writes that Hahnemann's disciples are encouraged to meditate on the book, paragraph by paragraph, in order to grasp the spirit of it. Dr J Kunzil confirms this:

'You all know that today we are witnessing a reinstatement and new progressive emergence of homoeopathy in many countries. This entire movement will only lead to results on condition that it draws its strength exclusively from the *Organ*... A dry, historical and theoretical study will serve no purpose and will bring no help to your patients. You've got to penetrate the spirit of this remarkable book; you must reflect and meditate on all it contains, and the more you study it, the greater will be the profit you'll derive from it.' ★

The President of the International League on Homoeopathy, a doctor from Rome, chose words at the Montreux Congress that make the position clear to a discerning Christian: 'It's futile to reject this or that principle enunciated in the *Organ*. There remains more than enough to recognise the unfathomable intuition and divinatory spirit of its author.'

Hahnemann and the *Organ*

The picture of Hahnemann presented by Trevor Cook in his biography *Samuel Hahnemann* is that of a religious freethinker, decidedly deistic rather than Christian, and a freemason. He was described as a godly man, at least according to the traditions of his day. He practised mesmerism, a kind of hypnosis assumed by Mesmer to be based upon the occult radiation of power.

Hahnemann placed on the title page of his *Organ* the words *aude sapere* (dare to be wise) the freemasonry motto.

In the *Organ* we read: 'A person becomes ill when a diseased agent infiltrates the body and disturbs the vital energy by dynamistic influence.' So what is this 'vital energy'? Man is body, soul (mind, will and emotions) and spirit. Hahnemann's concept of spirit was 'vital energy', the Hindu 'prana'. Like so many therapies in this area of alternative medicine, homoeopathy is a spiritual treatment, and accordingly the cure is applied *to* this vital energy. Also the law of similarity (or homoeo-

★ *Swiss periodical Journal on Homoeopathy* - No 2/1962.

pathic magic) provided for in the *Organ* means that the cure must resemble the disease as closely as possible in the totality of its symptoms when tested on a healthy man. The *Organ* states: 'All homoeopathic medicines cure illnesses the symptoms of which they most resemble.'

The *Organ* has this to say about this 'immaterial energy' or 'vital energy': 'The doctor can only remove these morbid affections (illnesses) by bringing to bear on this immaterial energy certain substances endowed with modifying properties that are equally immaterial (dynamic) and are discerned by the all-pervasive nervous system. Accordingly it's only by their dynamic action on the vital energy that the curative remedies are able to redress and do indeed redress the biological balance and restore health.'

The 'prana' of yogic philosophy, the 'innate' energy described by Palmer, the founder of chiropractic, the 'ch'i' from China, the 'force' that many traditions see as God, and the 'vital energy' of the homoeopathic doctors; are they not all pure deception? On from homoeopathy, Rudolf Steiner took the same concept and gave us anthroposophical treatments. They are generally homoeopathic containing the same occult force.

Of course those who see some sort of scientific or even natural energy at work in water divining, or who believe that water divination is a gift from God, will perhaps have some difficulty in seeing the evil that is at work in homoeopathy.

Power through diluting and shaking

Homoeopathic preparations may be sweetened or given a taste, but diluting and shaking using quite ordinary water is the essence of the idea. The teaching is that the more diluted the substance, the more powerful it is. Dilution is measured according to a scale from CH 1 to CH 100, or more, and each of the dilutions from 1 to 100 is made according to one drop of the previous dilution plus ninety-nine drops of water or liquid. Dr Bopp tells us that

...any patient receiving a homoeopathic treatment at CH 30 should be under no illusions as to its composition. There is no longer any material substance in the pill or liquid whatsoever. However, such mathematical proof doesn't in the least upset the homoeopathic doctors. Their teaching declares that the more diluted the substance, the more active it is. It's not just a question - and this is their secret - of a simple dilution, but of a process known as dynamisation or potentialisation, produced by repeatedly shaking the mixture between dilutions. Such repeated concussion makes it possible to contact and retain a hidden power in the liquid, its immaterial essence.

What does the British Medical Association (BMA) have to say?

It could not be expected that the working party of medical scientists, however distinguished, reporting in May 1986 would be able to discern the 'immaterial essence' known to the homoeopaths and which Dr Bopp refers to, nor to admit the possibility of any immaterial force at work. However their report, whilst evidencing disbelief in the involvement of what are in fact demonic forces, presents a useful opportunity to read a considered orthodox medical view. They write this:

"No pharmacological basis for homoeopathic

therapeutics could be found in the administration of a few drops of concentrations of remedies so dilute that a concentration of 12C, for example, may no longer contain one molecule of the original remedy, but will contain many different molecules of the fluids or powders used to dilute the original remedy. Nor indeed was any pharmacological basis claimed by individuals who discussed homoeopathy with the working party. What was claimed by the originator and is still claimed today, is that the process of dilution and 'succussion' effects an 'immaterial and vital' force and that this force is therapeutic. We have found no evidence for this belief." ★

The doctors balance that negative view with a recognition of the placebo effect known to all branches of medicine:

"…it appears that a placebo effect is the explanation of the belief, shared by homoeopaths and their patients, in the efficacy of homoeopathic therapeutics." ★

What about vaccination?

To the layman, vaccination and homoeopathy may seem to have much in common. Dr Bopp explains that in fact vaccination is quite different: 'Vaccination immunises an individual against a microbial disease by inoculating him with the attenuated microbe or its toxin. The technique is well known, clearly defined. It consists of stimulating the production of specific antibodies to act

★ *Alternative Therapy - Report of the Board of Science and Education* British Medical Association - May 1986).

against the microbe. Homoeopathy is not based on this technique. There is no production of specific antibodies.'

All homoeopathy is dangerous

Satan's lie is at the heart of all that is occult, and it is clearly seen in homoeopathy. As Dr Bopp puts it, the predominant strain of pantheism would place God everywhere, in each person, each animal, plant, flower, cell, and even in homoeopathic medicine. One homoeopathic doctor saw the role of his medicament in this way: 'The cure alone really knows the patient, better than the doctor, better than the patient himself. It knows just where to locate the originating cause of the disorder and the method of getting to it. Neither the patient nor the doctor has much wisdom or knowledge.' The doctor is really saying that the medicament has become a god.

Despite the fact that many Christians are being deceived and are turning from drugs to homoeopathy, it is another counterfeit — subtle, powerful and rooted in the occult. There can be no half measures. *All* homoeopathic and anthroposophical treatments have to be avoided.

Dr Bopp's conclusion, which could be applied with some slight variation to the great majority of therapies in this book, is as follows:

> … the occult influence, by nature hidden, disguised, often dissimulated behind a parascientific theory, does not disappear and does not happen to be rendered harmless by the mere fact of a superficial approach contenting itself simply with denying its existence. HOMOEOPATHY IS DANGEROUS. It is quite contrary to the teaching of the Word of God. It willingly favours healing through substances made dynamic, that is to say, charged with occult forces.

Homoeopathic treatment is the fruit of a philosophy and religion that are at the same time Hinduistic, pantheistic and esoteric. ... Contact with immaterial essence, the invisible force of the ethereal world operative in the medicament, sullies the Christian. The occult influence in homoeopathy is transmitted to the individual, bringing him consciously or unconsciously under demonic influence. Very often the result is a bond with Satan. A person may be cured of a bodily ailment... but spiritual life ebbs away. In this very connection it is significant frequently to find nervous depression in families using homoeopathic treatments.

Christians must not allow themselves to be seduced by the fact that homoeopathy can effect remarkable cures. It's not a question of denying them, even if scientific medicine lacks the explanations. The Bible teaches us that Satan, through the agency of men, is capable of performing miracles and healings. *'For there shall arise false Christs, and false prophets, and shall shew great signs and wonders; insomuch that, if it were possible, they shall deceive the very elect'* (Matthew 24:24).

Kentian homoeopathy - the deception deepens

Dr Charles Elliott in an article in 'Homoeopathy' Journal (Sept-Oct 1978) reminds us of how the higher potencies (or dilutions) are viewed by homoeopathic doctors. He writes: "The medicines, *non material at their higher potencies,* work quickly..." (emphasis mine). In other words at the material level and after much dilution the substance and the water has resulted in pure water; at the non-material level — in the spiritual realm — the medicine becomes quickly effective.

In 1980 Dr Elliott succeeded Dr Margery Blackie as

the Royal homoeopath. Both these doctors; like Sir John Weir before them, come from the particular wing of the homoeopathic discipline known as Kentian after an American homoeopath, James Tyler Kent (1849-1916). This is homoeopathy in its most extreme metaphysical form. "Kent had been one of the first to paint word pictures, indicating the kind of personality which matched a particular medicine. These word pictures now become central to homoeopathy. Through links with a form of Spiritualism called Swedenborgianism, they showed that its practitioners believed homoeopathy to be divinely revealed... On one level, it seems to have descended from the 'doctrine of signatures', as endorsed by Paracelsus - the very figure whose principles were recommended to BMA doctors by Prince Charles in December, 1982. The doctrine claimed that plants and herbs revealed by their appearance the medical purpose for which Nature had designed them: yellow plants for jaundice, heart-shaped leaves for heart complaints." ★

"Such a belief required a fundamental underpinning, one which argued that there was a divine force administering the harmony between man and nature. Again, Paracelsus anticipated homoeopathy by claiming the potency of remedies was spiritual rather than bio-chemical and that minute doses could combat major diseases." ★

What can be discerned from the writings of the homoeopath authorities can be confirmed by the experience of Christians. An adminstrator in the Faculty of Homoeopathy testifies in this way:

"As a Christian, one recognises the two sides of the spiritual realm - the good and the evil. .... In homoeo-pathy, you are definitely into the spiritual realm. It is very easy to make a religion out of it. ... If one reads Hahnemann's own writings, it's very easy to treat it like the Bible and end up in a state of worshipping Hahnemann and homoeopathy. I've seen it happen. It takes over. Without a shadow of doubt, nearly all the doctors attending the faculty are involved in some sort of spiritual practice — anthroposophy, transcendental meditation. Two doctors who were seeking recruits to Scientology set up practice using homoeopathy to attract patients to them. I believe in homoeopathy but I also believe it has an evil and dangerous side to it if is administered for the wrong purpose." ★

That is an interesting testimony from one who is acquainted with many who practise homoeopathy but it must be emphasised again that *all* homoeopathy, like all Satan's wiles, is dangerous. As a searcher in the area of occult healing I never met a practitioner who didn't believe that *some* spirits were evil. But they didn't know which. Apart from the Holy Spirit neither they nor I *could* know which. We didn't know that Satan could masquerade as an angel of light. Involvement with homoeopathy, like any involvement in this counterfiet spiritual realm, leads to further and deeper involvement, and, apart from the grace of God, to still further confusion and blindness.

That is the position of many Christians today. We need to separate ourselves from involvement with these occult deceptions. We need to renounce them and repent of our involvement with them asking the Lord to lead us into all truth.

★   *The Prince and The Paranormal*

Discernment, the Test of Scripture and our Intellect

With this detailed chapter on homoeopathy we conclude the chapters drawing attention to particular alternative therapies.

Deuteronomy 18:10-11 is a most significant scripture against which to consider any alternative medicine:

> *'There shall not be found among you any one that maketh his son or his daughter to pass through the fire, or that useth divination, or an observer of times, or an enchanter, or a witch, or a charmer, or a consulter with familiar spirits, or a wizard, or a necromancer.'*

Discernment comes by comparing to all of God's word and through the gift of the ability to distinguish between spirits (1 Corinthians 12:10).

In an article about homoeopathy in the Nurses Christian Fellowship magazine, 'Pacemaker', General practitioner Dr Andrew Fergusson applied to homoeopathy tests suggested by Christian Szurko to a Christian Medical Fellowship Study Group looking into alternative medicine. These tests were listed in Chapter Three. We are certainly not to discard our intellect in reckoning these matters, and the first five tests applied by Dr Fergusson to homoeopathy, seen in the following extracts, may usefully be applied to other therapies also. Before applying the five tests, Dr Fergusson identifies the three main principles in homoeopathy:

"1. The similia principle - 'like cures like'. Substances which ingested produce symptoms like those of the disease will cure that disease.

2. Increasing potency of preparations is achieved by increasing dilutions to produce infinitesimally small doses. Solutions of the allegedly therapeutic substances

are repeatedly diluted either 1 to 10 or 1 to 100 (on the X and C scales respectively), so that those preparations alleged by homoeopaths to be most potent in fact have no molecules of the original substance in them at all, and any efficacy comes from another source, usually claimed to be the 'energy' imparted in shaking or 'succussing' between dilutions.

3. The treatment is individualised to the patient after a lengthy history covering many aspects of the patient, and a detailed holistic approach is taken to the patient rather than to a single disease process..."

Having identified the three principles in homoeopathy we can now see how Dr Fergusson applies the tests:

"1. Do the claims made for it fit the facts?

Homoeopaths are reluctant to make any claims for efficacy which are objectively verifiable. References in generally accepted, peer-reviewed, medical literature can be counted on the fingers, if not thumbs, of one hand, and homoeopathic literature is anecdotal or contains reports of research which do not satisfy scientifically accepted double-blind controlled trial criteria. However, attempts are being made to apply the methods of acceptable scientific validation to homoeopathy, but the nature of their subject makes this difficult.

Care is taken to avoid making any claims which might be tested in court. For example, a statement of their own★ on homoeopathic pertussis vaccines reads: 'There is a lack of acceptable evidence that these vaccines provide effective protection.' It is at least likely that any improvement on homoeopathic treatment comes from placebo effects, homoeopaths' own claims of 30-40%

★ Faculty of Homoeopathy in Pharmaceutical Journal 14.12.85 p.773.

successes being around the usual placebo response. It is accepted that, especially in comparison with allopathic treatments, the preparations are usually not physically harmful. (This may not be unconnected with the fact that there is often nothing there — at least, nothing material).

There are no facts and homoeopaths are cautious in their claims.

2. Is there a rational scientific basis to the therapy?
The author can find no rational scientific basis to the first two principles outlined above. The whole person approach of the third principle is accepted by most good doctors nowadays.

3. Is it the methodology or is it the principle which is the effective element?
The author can find no proof of objective effect. The principles seem hard to relate to twentieth century scientific understanding, and methodology varies from practitioner to practitioner such that treatments are never comparable.

4. What are the assumptions of the world view behind the therapy?
It is said there are none, but the mystical 'energy' and 'vital-force' concepts smack of Hinduism. Hahnemann was a freemason, a mesmeriser, and a deist rather than a Christian. Christian homoeopaths admit these facts about their founder but are not concerned. Although most Christians would surely be worried by the philosophical and religious beliefs implicit and explicit in Hahnemann's writing, it must be remembered that by the medical standards of his day he was an enlightened and humane practitioner, in the physical sense. Whether his own religious beliefs should concern present day practitioners is a matter for individual decision.

5. Does the therapy involve the occult?

Leading Christian homoeopathic physicians have conceded to the author in personal communication that they know of some practitioners who use occult practices specifically forbidden in Scripture as part of their art.

"The author would submit that homoeopathy overwhelmingly fails the... five tests and, philosophically at least, must therefore be in no way from God but from the Devil who is 'a liar and the father of all lies.' (John 8 v 44). The author could not recommend any Christian to receive homoeopathic treatment or practise homoeopathic medicine, and believes that God is increasingly opening eyes to the pitfalls of this subject.... .

However, may the debate continue in that spirit of love and light which characterises the Lord, and not in the spirit of heat and darkness which seems to reflect the other place!" ★

Indeed may the debate continue among Christians. May we be open to hear one another. Above all may we be open to hear what the Holy Spirit is saying to us. And may we ever remember to check all things with Him and with the Word.

Any move away from Scripture can be a move in the direction of the *occult*. Another doctrine can become another gospel. As men have followed men apart from the leading of the Lord, *cults* have been born.

★ Article in *Pacemaker* by Andrew Fergusson The Journal of the Nurses Christian Fellowship (December 1987).

10
Cults and the occult
- a checklist

God's word in Deuteronomy (18:9-14) and in other Scriptures, forbids involvement in the occult realm. The answer to involvement is in renunciation, repentance and faith in Jesus Christ and His atoning blood. The help of Bible-believing, born again Christians is also needed by those deeply affected. Through them the powers of Satan can be rebuked and deliverance brought in the name of Jesus.

Before release will come it is often necessary for Christians to pray in the name of Jesus that the Holy Spirit will bring to their minds an honest and truthful recollection of past occult involvements. The names of therapies highlighted in the previous chapters may serve as reminders for this.

The checklist that follows includes broad areas of cults and the occult. They are arranged in no significant order and the names are once again intended to assist in the recall of past involvement. Some areas are covered more than once where different names are used. Some are already referenced in the body of the book as alternative medicine therapies. Others are difficult to categorise in one section or another. However they can all have a common source and there can be an occult element with each of them. Some of the items listed will have a harmless or even Christian application. An example is the sort of 'handwriting analysis' used by the police; this is perfectly acceptable. Another that is listed is 'exorcism'. This is another word for deliverance; the counterfeit of Christian deliverance or exorcism is practised by some who use occult power. Another example is tongues.

The list is not intended as a basis for further research or to throw at unsuspecting Christians unfamiliar with the sort of message that is central in this book. We have all of us, in some measure, been open to some of Satan's wiles. The Holy Spirit will be the communicator and if He can use this list to prompt a reminder of a past involvement that needs renouncing, then it will have served its purpose. Frequently too, the mention of one area can prompt the recall of others not listed or described in the same way.

The Bible tells us (Exodus 20:5, Deuteronomy 23:2, etc) that the sins of our fathers are carried through to future generations. The checklist can serve to remind of any known involvements by past or present members of the family. It is right to renounce our involvement no matter how innocently, even once, and at whatever age. Satan is no respecter of age or of persons. We are born sinners and Satan knows it! We need to consider if at any time we were present when things listed were going on. In these days it is also necessary to consider our openness to occult areas through radio and TV as well as through books, school, films, etc. There is no need to struggle and agonise over what is after all, a formidable list. As we look carefully through, we can trust the Holy Spirit to bring recall if we approach it in a prayerful way from the heart; also God can give discernment to others for us.

Occult

Hatha Yoga	Magic (black & white)
Cartomancy	Reincarnation
Fortune telling	Spiritism

Palmistry
Charms
Birth signs
Pentagrams
Ouija boards
Levitation
Automatic writing
Clairvoyance
Clairaudience
Divination
Telepathy
Superstitions
Mind control
Psychic powers
Pendulum swinging
Table tipping
Handwriting analysis
Hallowe'en
Akashic records
Almanac
Age of Aquarius
Aquarian gospel
Soul travel
Horoscopes
Atlantis
Aura
Taboos
Amulets
Dream interpretation
Exorcism
ESP
Rudolf Steiner
Intuitive arts counselling
Phrenology
Card cutting
Hand reading
Teacup reading

Tarot cards
Spells
Hypnosis
Osiris
'Dungeons and Dragons'
Astral travel
Taekwondo
Taoism
Mushindo karate
Aikido
T'ai Chi Ch'uan
Karate
Hapkido
Wu Shu
Spirit combat
Feng-sao
Dowsing
Soothsayers
Augury
Automatic drawing
Devil Dancing
Fetishes
Firewalking
Hexagrams
Omens
Telekinesis
Mesmerism
Autosuggestion
Cabbala
Mascots
Numerology
Incantations
Talismans
Fantasy role-playing
  games
Card reading
Psychoanalysis

Rod divination
Seances
Martial arts
Judo
Ju-jitsu
Ch'uan-fa
Kung-fu
Weeping Statues
Standing stones
Ley lines
Religious idols
Church pagan connections
Graphology
Incubus
Succubus
Parapsychology
Psycho-cybernetics
UFO's
Yoga
Charming
Curses (*by* you or *on* you)
Lucky charms
Kabala
Tribal dancing
Astral projection
Candle staring
Drugs
Ghosts
Pagan celebrations
Gipsy curse
Psychokinesis (PK)
Zodiac signs
I Ching
Moving Statues

Freud
'Holy' objects
AMORC
Oriental ornaments
Addictions
Spoon bending
Voices in the mind
Tongues (counterfeit)
Evil eye
Electric shock treatment
Nanbudo
Water divining
Mirror mantic
Kissing of idols
Glass moving
Idols
Teraphims
Stargazing
Old Moore
Stonehenge
Demonised souvenirs
Buddhas
Swastika
Images (frogs, cats, owls, bats and night creatures used in witchcraft)
Indian elephants
Pyramids
Obelisks
Serpents
Witch markings
Myths
Fairies and pixies
Mass (unbiblical)

Cults

Anglo-Israelism
The Worldwide Church
  of God
Baha'ism
Black Muslims
Christian Science
Conceptology
Freemasons and other
  secret societies
I AM
Inner Peace Movement
Lourdes
Madonna and Child
Spiritualism
Swedenborgianism
Theosophical Society
Unitarianism
Unity School of
  Christianity
Universalism
Ultimate reconciliation
Voodoo
Witchcraft
Zen Buddhism
Marxism
Moral Rearmament
Astrology
Human Potential
  Movement
Children of God
Hare Krishna
Gurdjieff
Baba-lovers
Sufi

Jehovah's Witnesses
Modernism, liberalism
  and the social gospel
Mormonism
New Thought
Rosicrucianism
Satanism
Scientology
Seventh Day Adventism
Spiritual Frontiers
  Fellowship
Saints
Medugorje
Communism
Buffaloes
Islam (Mohammedism)
Hinduism
Buddhism
Humanism
Eastern ceremonial dances
Pagan customs
Shrines
Pagan tourist places
Subud
Shepherding/Discipleship
Moonies
Unification Church
Anthroposophy
'Star Wars'
Theosophy
False philosophies
Belief systems
Mary worship
Eckankar

Transcendental Meditation	Est
	The Way
Divine Light Mission	Personal growth movement
Christadelphianism	Mind dynamics
The Healing Movement	Erhard Seminars Training
Cooneyites	The Aquarian Gospel
False religions	Zoroastrianism
Druids	Family of Love
Fatima	Walsingham
Roman Catholicism	

That is a formidable list of areas that *can*, in one way or another, open the way for Satan. Let us not take a wholly intellectual viewpoint and trouble ourselves unduly about whether a particular area is properly defined there as a cult or as occult. Items could have been omitted in order to satisfy the intellectual mind! However I believe this would have made the list less useful.

11
Sorting out the alternatives!

Language fails!

I have tried to slot each therapy into a broad category (physical, psychological and paranormal therapies, and paranormal diagnosis). I have tried in the last chapter to separate the cults and the occult. The distinctions are necessarily broad ones. When we look at therapies that emphasise the occult and therapies that emphasise psychology or a misplaced faith, we once again find difficulty. There is no clear dividing line. Christians will accept or reject a therapy for themselves according to the leading of the Holy Spirit.

At one end of the danger scale, spiritual healing is occult and mightily dangerous, as I learned through my own experience. It is forbidden according to God's word. At the other end of the scale there are the innocuous treatments; Christians can teach that God's way is even better. In between, we find therapies like homoeopathy, discussed in Chapter Nine. Apart from its root in the occult we have seen that its power is based upon the deception of energy passing from the herb or mineral into the water, in line with traditional Hindu beliefs. Also in homoeopathy there is room for the 'faith' element, of the placebo kind, that will help the success of the treatment along in the same way that many orthodox drugs are made more effective. Not so obviously perilous, but quite unlike the kind of faith we can receive from God, and unlike the leaves provided for our healing (Ezekiel 47:12), are those therapies involving a faith in some fantasy that has no basis in scripture or in science. The inert placebo★ is the best example.

Our relationship with Jesus starts with our coming to Him and receiving Him in *faith* (John 1:12). Our walk with Jesus is a walk in faith. *'So then faith cometh by hearing, and hearing by the word of God'* (Romans 10:17). The sort of faith we *actually* have is mirrored either by the depth of our descent into Satan's kingdom or by the heights to which we trust God to lead us. Jesus can meet health and healing needs. We can receive from Him as we get more and more revelation of the truth that is in Scripture.

Language cannot easily describe divine healing, simple though it is, to a disbelieving world. The same is often true when it comes to explaining occult alternative medicine, even to a Christian. I have walked with Satan into meditation, yoga, spiritual healing, divination with the pendulum, biofeedback, and more besides. I have walked with God in the power of the Holy Spirit. These are two different realms, one is the counterfeit of the other, but both are in a dimension different to the one the world knows. Language fails, but the truth is in God's supernatural word — the Bible.

In looking at alternative medicine we have to beware the irrelevant questions. On the world's view, any question is a fair question. We can sometimes be taken by a skilled debater to a point where we are cornered. Language is an even greater problem when we describe

★ The 'inert' placebo can be something like a sugar pill that can have no medical effect. However doctors usually prescribe what might well be called the 'deceptive' placebo - a pill designed to perform some function, albeit irrelevant to the patient's need.

136

the spritiual dimension. Satan is a master with words and he can deceive us with them. Given an opportunity, he will work through our intellect. 'This therapy is really only for relaxation, isn't it?'; 'Now you're not really worshipping me when you're only doing it for exercise, are you?'; 'Oh, we both know Charlie well. You're not suggesting he's not really a Christian, are you?'; 'What's the harm in meditation; Christians do it, don't they?'; *'Ye shall not surely die: For God doth know that in the day ye eat thereof, then your eyes shall be opened, and ye shall be as gods, knowing good and evil.'* (Genesis 3:4-5).

The Bible tells us that Satan only comes to kill and steal and destroy, and in the Garden of Eden the serpent stole from Eve the truth of God's word. It has been happening ever since. The serpent's lie was subtle and complex in the garden. It is subtle and complex in Hinduism, and that subtlety is perceivable in the same way in alternative medicine. Hinduism is not against any other religion. Alternative medicine and its practitioners are not against any other form of medical treatment. They focus directly on the question, 'Does it work?', mostly blissfully unaware of Satan masquerading as an angel of light.

The language of Hinduism

All is one! The natural; the supernatural; Satan; God; man; animals; the earth; life; death; the Creator; the creation. The Hindu sees the whole physical world, including sickness and health, as an illusion (maya). Is it surprising that the value placed upon life is so low in the Hindu lands? The Hindu sees everything as a unity developing through 'evolution' to 'enlightenment'. The idea of evolution was essential to Hinduism long before Darwin came along and grabbed the limelight. Indeed, evolution ideas were essential to Hinduism *and* Buddhism; also to Taoism which is a blend of these with Confucianism, and more, added. The Hindu doctrines added together promote the lie that man is God who doesn't need salvation from his sin. I myself had a guru (a Hindu spiritual teacher). I so trusted him that no objective argument could have pulled me from the path to the 'enlightenment' he was bringing me into.

Biofeedback was the principal tool I used as I learned from my guru. Once I accepted that the altered state of consciousness I was reaching was 'higher', I came to see the everyday experiences of life as being 'lower', nothing but *maya* compared to the real experiences I had come into, and the enlightenment I had started to look forward to. I didn't know this was all deception. I didn't sit around philosophising either! I was above all that, and 'experience' was the great thing! Really, I was enjoying the experiences. I didn't know the intellectual explanations. I didn't know that my eventual enlightenment was supposed to come with the experience of the 'atman' (or individual soul) being at one with the 'Brahman' (the universal soul) and when I would see myself as God! Neither did I know that the Holy Spirit who indwells Christians would come and dwell in me if I asked the resurrected Jesus into my life.

One Christian writer★ postulated Satan's system of logic in this way: 'God could not create something from nothing; therefore everything must be part of God; since God cannot be divided into parts, then everything is God and God is everything.' By the end of my 'search' into alternative medicine I was blinded by this sort of logic and I was a Hindu. I didn't call myself a Hindu; few Hindus do. Hinduism is a religion quite special to the Antichrist. Apart from occult healing, the other things I

★ *Peace Prosperity and the Coming Holocaust* by Dave Hunt - Harvest House, USA (1983).

138

was into also focused on Hinduism; all the Lord has shown me since reveals more about Hinduism. It is promoted everywhere, but it's not called Hinduism!

As a searcher, I prayed to an Indian god. He is alive today, a human being with an earthly body. As a serious searcher I found the god who is said, even by Christian writers, to be perhaps the most powerful psychic in the world today. My experience of this man was both on film at a private viewing in a London basement, and at a shrine on the outskirts of London. Also his presence was manifested to me on a London railway station. Without hesitation I can say he is a man capable of tremendous miracles, but he is deceived, and I was deceived. The miracles were counterfeit. However, they were still miracles. They are done in the power of Satan as if by a man walking in the flesh, as the antichrist in the flesh will one day do them. They are not some sort of conjuring trick as I have heard some mature Christians suggest. Christians need to grasp - contradictory though it may sound - the power and reality of counterfeit miracles. They also have to grasp the nature of the spiritual power, and the significance of the results that are achieved, in occult alternative medicine.

A ten pound note can be counterfeited. It can, through the quality of the deception, present a real challenge to the Bank of England. It can perhaps circulate for years before it is discovered. So it can be with Satan's deceptions! The note is not an illusion nor a theatrical conjuring trick; it circulates just like a real note. Some of these notes might even be the same as the real notes. All they lack is the authority of the bank.

Counterfeit healing miracles really do happen. I was miraculously cleared of a complaint that had troubled me daily for eighteen years. The power of Satan to remove symptoms is not an illusion. It is a biblical truth. Matthew 24:24 speaks of false Christs and false prophets, in the *plural*: 'For there shall arise false Christs,* *and false prophets, and shall show great signs and wonders; insomuch that, if it were possible, they shall deceive the very elect.'*

Surely we can see that happening in these days, but with the truth in our hearts we can take our minds off the question, 'Does it work?' and be open to receive discernment as to the source.

According to the prevailing thought in western society, the surest way to unpopularity is to appear critical of the ways of others. 'Live and let live!' is a popular phrase. The churchman might misrepresent Matthew 7:1 *'Judge not, that ye be not judged'.* Many a hippie 'did his own thing', took the drug trail to Northern India and Nepal, and ended up in hell. The Bible way is that we should look out for one another. The Hindu doctrine, having no problem with apparent contradictions, is that each person has to discover his own code of conduct. This doctrine of 'dharma' is with us in the West; it might aptly be called 'live and let die'.

The Hindu way of accepting all other religions invites an inevitable difficulty for the Bible-believing Christian. He loves the Hindu but, unlike the rest, he cannot accommodate his religion. Christians believe in the reality of an eternal life in heaven or in hell. The Hindu belief is in reincarnation and in the impersonal force that is in everything. The Hindus in the East, and their unknowing disciples in the West, still need to hear from Bible-believers of the reality of the Creator and living God.

The truth is in the Bible where it says, *'All scripture is given by inspiration of God'* (2 Tim 3:16). Both Hinduism and occult medicine are detestable to the Lord (Deuteronomy 18:10-12). After the serpent's lie came the fall of man. Whatever the serpent said, Eve *was* going to die spiritually. What the serpent said made sense according to Eve's thinking, and the serpent's lies are believed by the world today.

Alternative medicine, and this all-embracing religion of Hinduism which pervades so much of it, are the weapons Satan is using today to bring spiritual death. See how the logic ran in the Garden of Eden. You shall not surely die. You will be like God. By persuading Eve to eat of the tree of knowledge, Satan implied that this knowledge (the 'enlightenment' or 'cosmic consciousness' of the occultists) was the key to godhood. Satan tries to persuade us that the universe, and all in it, is a self-existent unity rather than God's creation: 'How could any tree cause death if it grows out of the same ground as other trees that sustained life? All is one by virtue of the Force that is all and is in all.'

Increasingly the world is coming to the Hindu view that God is not separate from his creation. The lie of Eden that we shall not die is perpetuated by the Hindu belief in reincarnation. I believed in reincarnation until the day I asked Jesus Christ into my life. For me, as for so many others, this belief, rather than a belief in heaven and hell, was the inevitable result of my progress in occult alternative medicine. The lie of Eden, that we shall be like God, reflects the Hindu view that all is one, with its echo that we are all God.

Those who attempt healing in the spiritual realm are inviting demons to manifest counterfeits, unless they know Jesus and have the right to use His name. The implication that the tree of knowledge brings godhood seems justified when it is discovered that life's mysteries can be found by moving into a dimension once unknown. After discovering the counterfeit peace that comes from yoga, the modern-day housewife moves on. Eventually she may well experience 'astral projection' and feel herself leaving her body. For the Hindus, and those who do move on, there is the feeling of unity with all around them and with creation. They can become aware of energy flows through them and from them. They recognise a power which may lead them to lay hands on the sick, to contact the dead, to work magic, and so on. It's a complex deception from beginning to end. The dead are *not* contacted.

Spiritualists cite the Scripture (1 Samuel 28) where the witch of Endor brought up Samuel from the dead at the request of Saul. There are different interpretations of this text. Even Bible language can be difficult, but the Holy Spirit is available to quicken to us the truth of God's word. When, God, through His word, speaks terror into the lives of sinners, He will open a door of hope if they repent. However those that go running to the gates of hell for help in the manner of King Saul must expect to find darkness there without any shafts of light. If it is the case that God permitted the devil to deceive Saul, 'as one who refused to love the truth' (2 Thess 2:10-11), there is no way for spiritualists to get any comfort from it. Samuel and Saul lived under the old covenant, and another interpretation is based upon 1 Samuel 28:15: *'And Samuel said to Saul, why hast thou disquieted me, to bring me up?'* That was written in God's Word and so, it is interpreted, it *was* Samuel as the truth was there written and could not have been a demon speaking. Today's spiritualist mediums should however take no comfort from that. The situation was changed by the death of Jesus. Jesus *'And having spoiled principalities and powers, he made a show of them openly, triumphing over them in it'* (Colossians 2:15). Whatever power Satan may have had under the old covenant, Jesus took back the authority Satan had received through Adam's sin. On either popular interpretation of the witch of Endor scripture today, the dead are *never* contacted.

Language fails! But with the Bible we can have revelation; another lesson is clear from the witch's occult sin. The Bible doesn't describe the detail of *how* the witch 'brought up Samuel.' This is consistent with God's position in other Scriptures: *'For your obedience is come abroad unto all men. I am glad therefore on your behalf: but yet I would have you wise unto that which is good, and simple concerning evil'* (Romans 16:19), *But unto you I say, and unto the rest in Thyatira, as many as have not this doctrine, and which have not known the depths of Satan as they speak; I will put upon you none other burden.* (Revelation 2:24). The Scriptures are clear and they forbid our coveting to know 'Satan's so-called deep secrets.' Many Christians today, fired by the question 'Does it work?', are wanting to look deeper and deeper into what is occult alternative medicine. The Lord says to us today that He wants us to be 'innocent about what is evil.' We can receive God's discernment so that we may know what is of Him.

Of course Hindus, New Agers and occultists *do* work magic. The Bible says this is possible. However the occult medical magicians described in this book do not truly *heal* the sick. Satan gave Eve, and he gave Saul, a delusion. What we see in occult alternative medicine is a delusion of healing. Demons may take away the symptoms, but there is a worse physical, emotional or spiritual price to pay.

The pattern doesn't seem to vary much, and perhaps there is no reason to suppose Satan has any different outline plan for all the people. All who are being directed by Satan are on their way, whether they understand it or not, to that 'enlightenment' experience, which has many descriptions, and to eventual spiritual and eternal death. Meanwhile man, who is in Satan's grip in the area of the occult, will perhaps come to the position where a whole new world enfolds. If he is a scientist, he will see how the physical laws on which he had depended do not always apply; he will write 'new' science based upon his experience. If he has a mind to the health professions, he might become a powerful 'healer'. Through the steadfast working out of his original plan in the Garden of Eden,

Satan is seeing many in the West become powerful psychics.

A knowledge of Scripture is needed. God spoke through Hosea and said, *'my people are destroyed for lack of knowledge'* (Hosea 4:6). Paul told the Romans that the Israelites were zealous for God, *'...but not according to knowledge'* (Romans 10:2).

It is not so long ago that the only obvious expressions of Hinduism were confined to the drug-based spirituality of the hippie movement and to extraordinary trend setters like the Beatles with their venture into Transcendental Meditation. Satan takes Hindu evangelism very seriously! Who ever heard of a Hindu evangelist! They are in fact everywhere without knowing it; they have been dear to Satan's heart from the beginning! It has been described as a rich jungle that has grown and spread in tropical profusion.

Today we can see clearly how this oldest of religions is invading science and the arts. It is invading medicine and the church. In Chapter Fifteen a view is taken of the apostate church in Britian today. I believe there will be a coming together of the church and alternative medicine and with this I believe we shall see a reinforcement of the Hinduism to which both are open.

We take a further look at Hinduism in the next chapter, but first we look at the link which connects it into the New Age.

Hinduism and the New Age movement - the link

The Bible tells us that the man of lawlessness who is doomed to destruction will one day be revealed (2 Thessalonians 2:3). Christians describe this man as Antichrist who will come in the flesh. Hinduism has for long been preparing the ground and it is reasonable to believe that Antichrist, launching his New Age, will be doing so among people worldwide who have been made ready to accept him.

Constance Cumbey has made a study of the writings of Alice Bailey, and whilst we should be cautious with them because of their demonic source, many of them automatically written at the direction of a deceiving spirit known by Alice Bailey as The Tibetan, it is true that there can be found in these writings the guidelines followed by the New Age movement today. In particular Mrs Bailey wrote 'The Externalisation of the Hierarchy'; the general public were to be familiarised with the concept of the 'Hierarchy' and in 1946 she directed the New Age disciples to emphasise the following:

1.   The evolution of humanity and its goal of perfection. In other words men were to become as God, squarely in line with Hindu thought.

2.   The Relation of the individual soul to all souls. This is the idea that all-is-one, the doctrine of unity or interdependence of all of life. Once again this is a central doctrine in Hinduism.

3.   The belief in the spiritual Hierarchy will then be deduced; the normality of its existence will be emphasised. Along with this it would be taught that the 'Kingdom has always been present' though unrecognised.

4.   After the above three teachings have taken effect and become generally recognised, it will be emphasised that there are those who have already reached the goal of 'soul control.' In other words they would be possessed.

The idea was to be fostered amongst us that there are some so-called masters living in the flesh, and there follows the recognition that there would be one individual who had completed the evolutionary process. That individual would serve as head of the 'Hierarchy'. He would be 'Director of the Kingdom of God on Earth.'

In 'The Hidden Dangers of the Rainbow' ★ Constance Cumbey writes: "Other things were to be taught to prepare the world for the 'New Age' and the 'New Age Christ' as well ... New Age symbols such as the rainbow, Pegasus, the unicorn, the all-seeing-eye of freemasonry, and triple sixes were to be increasingly displayed ... Mind control and meditation were to be taught. Colour therapy was to be emphasised. Music therapy and holistic health were additional items to be added to the eclectic diet for a 'New Age'."

We know in the 1980s that Holistic Health, alternative medicine, IS part of the New Age diet!

We take note of Mrs Bailey and her New Age teaching just as we take note of Hitler and his occultic cohorts in order to come to an understanding of Nazism. However much as Mrs Bailey's work has fairly accurately served to describe the New Age this far - and the evidence is there to be checked - we may not assume that God will allow New Agers to continue to follow her teaching or to allow more of any New Age 'Plan' to come to pass. Also as Christians, accurate though the Bailey writings may appear to be, we are to take our revelation only from God's Word. We can know from the Bible that man is not to build the Kingdom on earth, that there is going to be no 'Director' except the King when He comes (1 Thessalonians 4:17), and that the signs of the end of the age are recorded there. (Matthew 24, Luke 21).

Yet we cannot escape the fact of the New Age movement, the fact that Holistic Health is part of the New Age and the evidence that New Age teaching today has its

★ Published by Huntington House Inc., Shreveport, Louisiana, USA - 1983.

root with Mrs Bailey. Beyond Alice Bailey we can go back further.

The New Age was not much in evidence as a movement until 1975. It then had permission from the Hierarchy, from the spirit guides, to go public. Yet the preparations had gone on for a long time before. The modern start was in 1875, the date of the founding of the Theosophical Society by Helena Blavatsky. There seems to be little doubt that Madame Blavatsky was the catalyst of the modern New Age movement and indeed the theology of the serpent in the Garden of Eden, unchanged through all generations, is the foundational truth of Theosophy. 'Theosophical Glossary'★ defines Theosophy as Divine Wisdom. The Hindu idea of reincarnation remained and expressed the lie of Genesis 3:4: *'Ye shall not surely die.'* The Hindu idea that man is a god became reflected in the lie that man was able by his own efforts to reach a new higher level of consciousness, the divine mind, or nirvana. Thus the New Agers follow also the lie of Genesis 3:5: *'ye shall be as gods.'* W Q Judge, one of the founders with Madame Blavatsky, has written of her:

"She wished all men to know that they are God in fact and that as men they must bear the burden of their own sins, for no one else can do it. Hence she brought forward to the West the old Eastern doctrines of Karma and reincarnation."★★

Madame Blavatsky left India in 1885, came to Europe and died in England in 1891. However the Theosophical Society was well established. She was followed by Annie Besant. Then came Alice Bailey, and the movement con-

★   Published by Los Angeles Theosophical Co.

★★ *H P Blavatsky* by W Q Judge (Los Angeles Theosophy Co.).

tinued, including through the important front organisations that exist today.

H G Wells is one among the famous who have involved themselves with Theosophy. Perhaps the least known, and certainly the most important of his books, is another 'bible' of the New Age. 'The Open Conspiracy' was first published in 1928 and in the Preface he writes, "This is my religion."

Jane Gumprecht thoroughly covers the New Age background in 'Holistic Health' and whilst these three ladies, Blavatsky, Besant and Bailey, cannot be separated from the Holistic Health story because of its relevance in the New Age 'Plan', one more very significant character is not left out. The Holistic movement was spawned not only by Blavatsky but also through Edgar Cayce (1877-1945), the American medium. The Bible says that Satan masquerades as an angel of light (2 Corinthians 11:14) and the achievements of Cayce in the area of psychic medicine are everywhere reported as truly remarkable. In line with the Theosophists he believed in reincarnation and karma; his philosophy of healing involved the attuning of the divine mind within to creative energies. His results were remarkable, like many today. Yet he was deceived for he knew not from whence the power came.

It is clear the New Age movement is not without its history, but now we come more up to date. We look briefly at the movement and some of the evidence today in the next chapter.

The scene for the decade of the 80s was set by Marilyn Ferguson in 'The Aquarian Conspiracy - Personal and Social Transformation in the 1980s'. Once again this is a well known and very significant book known to New Agers throughout the world. Deceived like the other ladies whose books serve as 'bibles' for the New Age movement, she is lacking in a knowledge of the truth, but nevertheless unmistaken in presenting the facts:

148

"For many Aquarian Conspirators, an involvement in
health care was a major stimulus to transformation.
Just as the search for self becomes a search for health
so the pursuit of health care leads to self-awareness.
All wholeness is the same. The proliferating holistic
health centres and networks have drawn many into the
concious movement." ★

As we look now at the New Age movement, let us not
doubt that the Holistic Health movement is a vital part of
it. It provides the most common and effective entree into
the Aquarian Conspiracy, the New Age. Satan seeks
control of our minds. As we have seen in the review of
therapies in Part Two, he can gain that control if we
allow him, whether through paranormal, psychological
or merely physical therapies.

★ *The Aquarian Conspiracy - Personal and Social Transformation in the 1980s* by Marilyn Ferguson. (1980) Grafton Books, -
A Division of Collins Publishing Group.

PART THREE
HEALING, THE CHURCH AND THE NEW AGE MOVEMENT

12
The New Age Movement

Satan's bride

Since writing the first two editions of this book I have made two journeys to America and travelled in that land with my eyes open! In Britain too, I believe the Holy Spirit is quickening us to what is even now little known among Bible-believing Christians — the New Age movement.

It is not a bureaucracy or an organisation but a network of social and spiritual movements. Each is self-sufficient. Not one of them is essential to the whole, but the New Age movement is becoming an evident source of potential power. The network is much greater than the sum of its parts.

Behind the New Age movement is Lucifer's desire to be worshipped as God. I believe that, as Jesus Christ prepares His bride (His Church), Satan prepares his counterfeit in the New Age movement. New Agers comprise many who have had their minds emptied by such practices as yoga, and who have come, or are coming, into a spiritual awareness in Satan's realm rather than in God's. They comprise also those who support social organisations, more worldly than spiritual, but which often evidence a marked denial of the teachings of Jesus. Often the organisations have an eminently respectable front. Then there are the seemingly endless movements concentrating on self and humanistic psychology. Many, if not all, are focusing on the creation.

Of course we should respect the creation, and some organisations which are intent on protecting it are in the New Age network which at this stage comprises both the spiritual and the worldly. They are bound together by their focus on the creation, whether set to discover the so-called deep secrets referred to in Revelation 2:24, or to preach about 'peace', mankind and looking after the creation.

New Agers will reach the end planned for them by many different routes — unless they turn to Jesus. They progressively find greater unity with one another, reaching their enlightenment in various ways hardly noticed by the world. The world knows the routes that are less obviously spiritual, like alcohol and rock music. Modern variations which Satan seeks to use to lead us to the same place have already been touched on in this book.

The rainbow

Individuals may realise they are part of a movement, or they may not. Even so, they attend the same festivals, read similar magazines and meet in the same vegetarian or health food establishments. More and more, both the New Agers 'exploring' the mysteries of the creation, and those wanting to 'protect' the creation, are found displaying the sign of the rainbow. They are familiar with the sign of the rainbow, and in the New Age it has its counterfeit meaning. It seems that in the New Age we have a movement that meets the scriptural description of the needs of the Antichrist and of the political movement that will bring him to power.

The rainbow is used to signal others in the network. They place them in their shops and motor-car windscreens. Christians seeing the symbol used in this way may well get witness in their spirit to discontinue using the sign themselves; it would be natural for the forces of darkness to encourage use among Christians, and what use is a symbol like this to those who are Christians? Some would say, "Why bother about a rainbow symbol? After all, it's God's symbol!" Some may say that, but God's sign to us is the *real* rainbow we see in the sky after the rain.

The New Age rainbow is a hypnotic device and New Agers call it an 'International Sign of Peace.' For them it signifies their building of a rainbow bridge between man and Lucifer, according to the spiritual tradition of the American Indians.

A newly-published children's story attracted my attention and excitement when, as a searcher, I was attending the World Assembly of Moral Rearmament in 1981. The story ends with an Indian grandfather telling his young grandson that the rainbow is a sign from 'Him who is in all things' that mankind is one big family. The youngster is encouraged to go to the top of the mountain, grow in the skills of manhood and learn to be a warrior of the rainbow, and to be one whose strong and obedient spirit will, through love, rise above the fear and hate in the world in order that destruction and war will be at an end.

The sign of the union of all people like one big family is a subtle deception and a twisting of God's truth. Whatever opposes God's truth is a lie. The lie is being promoted in different ways; today's New Agers are carrying on Satan's tradition. They are building a Rainbow Bridge, 'the antakarana', in the same way the Indians did, between Satan and mankind.

Many will remember the tragic sinking off New Zealand of the Greenpeace boat 'Rainbow Warrior'.

Doctrinally the ecology group Greenpeace looks to Red Indian legends. They look forward to a new tribe *'from all creeds'* who believe in deeds not words and who will restore the earth to its former beauty. The new tribe is one the Red Indians call the 'Warriors of the Rainbow'.

Blind to the Devil's devices one large evangelical Christian ministry, which had promoted products emblazoned with rainbows through a sizeable business operation, in 1986 ran a youth weekend called Vision Quest. The letter advertising this caught my attention because it showed a Red Indian in head dress with hand raised. I read that Vision Quest was a Red Indian term given to a time when a young brave goes out into the wilds alone and fasts for a number of days to seek for a vision to show what his new name is to be and give insight into his calling in life.

For those whom God has given eyes to see - spiritual eyes - there is ample evidence in these days that Christian ministries are really joining in spirit with New Agers to build the Rainbow Bridge between Satan and mankind. We saw this unity between Christians and New Agers, this time in the flesh also, at one large festival in 1986. This was a Christian gathering with leadership including that given to the rainbow and Vision Quest ventures referred to above. One principal speaker was the Director of another leading ecology group and he addressed several hundred of us with Another Gospel more akin to Earth Worship, not the Gospel of Jesus. Christians, however innocently, receiving Red Indian mythology from their leaders or a pantheistic message of earth worship from those they invite into fellowship, are in reality being led by the father of lies. It is not suprising when he who is controlling and ruling the whole world (1 John 5:17) plants a seed of deception based upon a scripture. However it is surely a sign of the times of the end when we contemplate the blatant invitation to Another Gospel given at that 1986 Christian Festival sponsored by several large covering ministries. Afterwards, while there was perhaps some heart searching prompted by a handful of protesters, the same Christian ministry that gave us Vision Quest and rainbows made available the cassette tape under its usual Christian label.

All deception in the Church has to be cut out wherever it is found if we are to contend for the faith as the Bible instructs us (Jude 3). Central to the deception is the idea of building the kingdom on earth. It is what Rome, the Jehovahs Witnesses and the other cults have for long been engaged in. Evangelical Christians are being drawn into the deception not only through identification with Rome, its ecumenism and syncretism well evident to most observers today, but also through identification with New Age groups like Greenpeace which also sees 'a tribe of people' *from all creeds* who will restore the earth to its former beauty. Through one way and another there are New Agers *and Christians* today who are building the kingdom here on earth.

These deceptions taken on board by evangelical Christians find their focus in building the kingdom on earth. In America it is being called 'Kingdom Now'. This is examined further in 'Understanding Deception - New Age Teaching in the Church'. In this book we look briefly at New Age healing deceptions in the church in Chapter Fifteen.

The stage is being set now

Networking groups are open to the idea of the same interconnecting 'force' or 'energy' given to eastern religions. Christians know that one day Antichrist will be revealed and we await the return of Jesus (2 Thessalonians 2: 1-3). Many of the new 'religious' New Agers we are seeing in the west, like the Hare Krishna people we see in our high streets, are often expecting the return of someone too. The Jews still await their Messiah. The Buddhists await the Fifth Budda. The Moslems await the Imam Mahdi. The Hindus await Krishna. No doubt the same Antichrist will satisfy them all, and may we not suppose that there will be professing Christians, deceived along the lines previously described, who are being brought to a place where they will be satisfied too?

On all fronts, pieces of the world jigsaw are fitting together and making a bigger and bigger network. The money system is near to collapse. A card payments system is ready to be brought in. There is increased use of '666', another of the symbols used by New Agers.

The stage for the Antichrist is being set now. Surely it is not in the nature of Satan's plan - and there is evidence in God's word - that the Antichrist will start his reign in the flesh as a sort of over-worked Secretary-General busily organising his troops and launching new symbols and brand names! The organisation has been built up over thousands of years! The scenario is there for those who have ears to hear (Revelation 13:9) and eyes to see. When the Antichrist is eventually known, doubtless the world will be ready to receive him. Will more and more see that this is in fulfillment of Bible prophesy, or will many be blinded to God's word? The world is happy to be served by 'great signs and miracles' performed by the false Christs in these days. How much more will the world be ready to receive and respect the miracles of the Antichrist when he is among us? Will the rainbow be ever more widely used across the world and be ready for the Antichrist to use as his own? Will it be seen that Satan could hardly have found a better symbol than the sign God gave to Noah, for his counterfeit in the New Age? Will Christians get more and more revelation of the end-time message from Scripture? Will Satan's counterfeits for the New Age become more and more credible, even as they become more obviously incredible to those who have eyes to see? Do Christians perceive that the revolution in occult medicine fits into Satan's greater design? Do we know, and do we have it clearly written in our hearts, that what is foretold in Scripture cannot fail to come to pass?

The New Age can only be recognised as such when compared to the reality found through the knowledge of the person of Jesus. The world has been ready for a lead. Biblical Christianity has always provided the answer. However, through the failure of our churches, it has been the New Age movement that seems to have come up with the solution. New Age leaders, unlike so many church leaders, have spoken clearly. It is the New Agers who have demonstrated the ways to change, whether from an immoral life-style to a more moral one, from denatured bread to the organic loaf, from consumerism to economic simplicity, from drugged childbirth to natural childbirth, from the excesses of modern medicine to individual healing 'of the whole person', and so on. These changes are good. The counterfeiter always starts with something good. On the evidence of what many are seeing to be clearly good, a wide cross section, from vegetarians to veterinarians, are being drawn into holistic health.

Blinded by science

We have been blinded by science for only a few generations. The wealth of the learning and research is stacking up all around us. It continues to be true that ninety per cent or more of all the scientists that ever lived are still alive today. Science goes further and further into specialisation. If a scientist has shown something to work, it has come to be called 'truth'. This applies to all science; of course medical science is no exception.

However, in these days, many scientists working in specialised disciplines are crossing over, not only into areas they don't understand, but also over the threshold into the areas of 'Satan's deep secrets' we read about in Revelation 2:24.

My own study of biofeedback and alpha waves was laid before me by scientists. The so-called scientific inventions of Kirlian photography and radionics, and the so-called discovery of biorhythms, and all the rest of the variations on the same occult deception, has taken scientists back into areas of knowledge practised by eastern mystics going back thousands of years. Throughout occult medicine and the rest of Satan's realm, modern man is putting scientific descriptions to the hidden knowledge that has been available since the fall of man to those who will turn from the truth.

I do not know where the line is drawn and where science ceases to be science. It is clear however that many scientists are deceived, and many of their 'discoveries' are deceptions from across the forbidden threshold. God will provide the discernment we each need in our own situations when we earnestly seek it. Similarly Satan will deceive us when we remain open to him.

'If it works, it is OK' is still the silent message that comes forth from the medical profession. Psychiatry too, is supposed to have a basis in science. I have heard of at least one psychiatrist converted to an eastern religion as a consequence of counselling a patient. Deception is stacked upon deception. How far this penetrates the scientific discoveries of the years' past may one day be revealed to us.

Computer networking

Computers appear to be scientific. Clearly they will be

significant as we move through the New Age. If there is no deception in them, then man can at least use them to deceive. The computer network will transfer and pass on deceptive information, broadcasting it at a speed not limited by time.

'Networking' is a New Age word. It is used wherever New Agers are to be found, and in July 1984 I visited the 'Networks 84' Computer Exhibition at the Wembley Conference Centre in London. Although I am a chartered accountant, there was little I could easily understand. As I moved from stand to stand I was at a loss to know how to start any sort of dialogue. The jargon was endless, making conversation very diffcult. I found occult symbols, such as pyramids, placed ornamentally in a manner of a vase or table lamp.

I attended the 'Mind-Body-Spirit Festival 84' at Olympia, London on the same day as the 'Networks 84' Exhibition. Here I learned more about Networking - the 'Peace Network' and 'Networking the Networks'. The Peace Network, according to the leaflet I was shown, was 'linking ideas, people and computers to build a more peaceful world.' The system of 'Networking the Networks' enabled those participating to feed information (people, places, resources, events) for the use of others, into the computer system. While the multinational corporations are having their needs met by computers, and whilst they are probably still in the forefront of computer applications, it is clear that costs have been so reduced, and applications made so flexible, that the information and communication, once the preserve of the wealthy, are now available to the ordinary folk who have a mind to change the world. Computers provide us with enormous benefits, but they will be enormously significant in the New Age. *'If any man have an ear, let him hear.'* (Revelation 13:9).

Beyond the social gospel

The world moves from one counterfeit to another, from the excesses of scientific medicine to holistic health care, from the consumer society and dead religion to the New Age and the powerful religion that lurks around the corner. Anyone who belongs to a church that offers only a short-changed spirituality will have no biblical standard against which to measure the wiles of Satan. Often it is a church itself, dynamic and alive, that leads its people, beyond the 'social gospel' so well known in the traditional church, taking them even further from a walk with the living God.

Typical groupings in the new age

As various ecology groups have sprung up in the New Age, it was inevitable that Christians would become involved. What we see is a focus on a oneness with each other and creation, on 'peace' and on what we find in nature. One group professes Christ, but New Age elements can be identified. Vegetarianism, the status of animals and the feminine role are subjects significant to them as they focus on what they see as God's 'Green World'. The world has no difficulty with that. Satan, the ruler of this world, will happily encourage it. As Christians we cannot take our eyes off Jesus; Satan is ready for the undiscerning. When we become dissatisfied with what we have, it is tempting to look around. There is no lack of provision as any 'searcher' will know well!

'The Christian Community' has centres across the world. It came about when another group of caring people felt the growing irrelevance of orthodox church life in meeting the disastrous events in world history and in understanding what they describe as the 'increasing complexities of man's inner experience.' Their search led them to Rudolf Steiner, the founder of Anthroposophical Medicine already referred to in Chapter Five. Through Steiner, we are told, a new approach to 'sacramental life' was given and 'The Christian Community will naturally turn to his work for inspiration and guidance.'★

Other communities have been established, some more avowedly Christian than others, committed variously to working for peace and justice, establishing radical lifestyles and to holistic medicine. Jesus died to give us a peace that passes all understanding; that is not the peace that the world seeks. Although the majority of these people are believed to be professing Christians, their movements have largely kept their commitment free of explicit reference to prayer and the Bible in order to make it possible for any person of goodwill to join in what they see as a matter of concern for the whole human family. Well-intentioned movements like these have stumbled into the New Age, often without realising it. Whilst they wouldn't want to be associated with occultism, Eastern religions or even Moral Rearmament, they occupy a significant place in the developing world view with eyes off the Creator but on the creation.

There is so much that could be valuable in these movements, but as things stand this is like the bait in a trap. Those who are feeling defeated or, like the founders and leaders of these movements, want to do something about the darkness that is upon the world, are looking for more than they see the world is able to give. However they can do nothing apart from knowing Jesus and turning to Him as their Saviour and Lord. It is the

★ *What is the Christian Community?* by Michael Tapp (Floris Books).

method of the ruler of this world to set the hearts of men on *anything* that will take their eyes off *Him*. Under the New Covenant, having received Jesus into our lives, we are New Creations in Christ Jesus and our bodies are the temples of the Holy Spirit. He wants to live our lives for us if we will let Him. He wants us to live by the power of the Holy Spirit. He wants to prove His sufficiency in every area of our lives. He wants us to join in the life of the community, but our ways are not His ways, and His ways are not man's ways.

The willing heart of the New Ager

When I was a New Ager I didn't give much thought to the particular churches I knew at that time. However, had I been comparing myself to many in the New Age and in these churches, the comparison would have been of two different extremes. The absence of life in the churches was to be contrasted with the New Age people who in one way or another were willing to spend hours each day in various efforts or arduous self-discipline. I was finding people who were starting life again, from scratch, building new life-styles away from consumerism and materialism, and who were, like the committed Christians I now know, prepared to bear without any hostility any derision that they received. They were deceived in spite of their efforts. However, had they turned to the churches that most of them knew, they would have found there no valid alternative.

The only answer is Jesus. Most New Agers, so often wanting to give so much, and so full of care for their fellow men, have never been in a place where they have heard the gospel of Jesus. Many had been regular churchgoers. Yet they never knew what Jesus himself said: *'Verily, verily, I say unto thee, except a man be born again, he cannot see the kingdom of God.'* (John 3:3)

They don't know that a new life-style is not the same thing. They don't know they are on a Hindu path, and that as they progress, they will be ever more blinded to the idea of being born again.

Hinduism: The predominant world view in the West ★

Two things make Hinduism deserving of at least a short section in any book dealing with aspects of the New Age:

1. Hinduism can accomodate any *religion* but it cannot accomodate Biblical Christianity.

2. The occult and New Age deceptions, including those found in Alternative Medicine, are substantially rooted in Hinduism.

At the intellectual level the religion is full of contradiction when viewed from a Western perspective. Sai Baba, perhaps the most powerful psychic in the world today, is styled by his followers as god, yet he acknowledges we are all gods. In puja rooms all over the world statues of Sai Baba are brought by his followers to be blessed by the manifestation of his sacred ash upon them. He is happy for statues of Jesus Christ to be taken to those same puja rooms to be blessed in a similar way. Satan and his demons are in control of the situation and the lie which they promote, and which runs through the Hindu rationale, is that God is part of His own creation. This is often expressed in the term - 'all is one'. All is god, and the whole creation hangs together by a 'force'. Hindu mystics and gurus have for long tuned into this

★ First appeared in *Understanding the New Age - Preparations for Antichrist's One World Government* (New Wine Press, 1986).

force and become aware of their 'godhood' and 'oneness' with the creation. Hinduism is significant in the New Age context because this monistic ('all is one') view of reality has progressively and quickly displaced Christanity as the world view predominant in the West. This is manifestly true when we look at alternative medicine and the branches of psychology at work in that and other areas, in science, in sociology and in education. Evolution, reincarnation and all the other aspects essential to Hinduism are found in the Religious Education taught in Western schools, where the Bible is an unknown book to vast numbers of youngsters.

Yoga classes are held everywhere in the West, and Yoga is Hindu. Self-realisation is its aim. Although it's not taught in the first course of lessons, and certainly even some teachers may not know it, the aim is to realise that we are gods. The class sits quietly in yoga positions. There is a stillness and a peace. There is a oneness. There comes a realisation that 'all is one'. Every yoga teacher is a Hindu missionary. Then there is a renewed interest in Sanskrit literature. The literature consists largely of hymns of praise and prayer, with sacrificial formulas and incantations as repeated by the priests. The Sanskrit literature is from India; it is in the sacred and ancient language of the Hindus.

Meditation of one sort and another, Transcendental Meditation, hypnosis and every variation can be found; they are really all the same and known to the yogis and gurus of the East for thousands of years. Their purpose in Satan's scheme is to bring a unity between Man and God - the abstract Hindu god who is really anybody and everybody. Yoga is a Hindu word which comes from the Sanskrit 'yo' and 'ga' - Man and God. The aim is for a unity such as is found by a drop of water when it falls into the sea. You can't find that drop of water anywhere. You believe you have become like God, but in fact you have lost your identity. The serpent lied when he encouraged Eve to question God and told her that she would never die. Satan is the liar in Hinduism too; there is no prospect of becoming like God, identity is lost. Soon everything can be lost if the Hindu way is followed.

My expectation as a Christian has nothing in common with Hinduism. I do not look forward any more to a reincarnation after death. Sai Baba, the god-man to whom I at one time prayed, is no answer for the souls who visit his ashram in their tens of thousands. He is a man deceived and possessed, perhaps like no other man alive today; he is a Hindu in India. My expectation is not of a merger with God to be all-one with Him. The promise that I have is that I shall see Him face to face. The distinction between me, a creature and God my Creator will always remain. I shall never become God. I shall never become equal to God. I shall never merge in Him. *There* lies the difference between Hinduism and Christianity.

What else does Hinduism teach? First there is reincarnation, the idea that after death we return to earth with another life. Hinduism teaches 'You will never die. You will become God.' The cruel lie of the serpent in Genesis 3:4 operates. Then there is karma, the idea that conditions in the next life are determined by those in the present one. What little incentive there is for the people to leave the streets of Calcutta even if they could. To help them would only serve to influence their karma for the next life. What we find among the most popular beliefs in the West in these days are little different; the issue is becoming a clear one. After looking at all the world's religions C S Lewis drew the conclusion there were just two possible choices: to become a Hindu or a Christian. The two don't mix. It is the choice we have, and those who choose the ways of the New Age choose Hinduism, the religion of the Antichrist.

13
From New-Ager to End-Timer

I didn't think of myself as a New Ager! Yet that is what I was. Apart from my involvement with alternative medicine, I belonged to many of the organisations that make up the New Age movement, that network of groups looked at briefly in the previous chapter that is unknowingly making the way ready for the one world ruler and the false prophet - the beast out of the sea and the beast out of the earth written about by John in the book of Revelation.

New Age and occult background

At the age of forty-three, my spiritual awakening began with a new awarenes of Moral Rearmament, and from there Satan took me into occult healing. In recent years I had been active in politics too, and at the time of my 'search' my political interests also took a significant turn. Before eventually resigning all the offices I held, I joined other organisations concerned with peace and justice. It was some time after my conversion that I could discern these as being really New Age organisations. It was much later still when I took a new view of my membership of these other organisations.

Now, outside of the political 'main line' where I had spent three years as a constituency party chairman, I was seeing a unity among groups. They were facing up to the nuclear and other threats to the creation and to personal freedom. That had become my New Age focus. I had not yet joined the body of Bible-believing Christians who were becoming increasingly aware that we must be in the end of the end times. As a non-religious individual, I was now identifying with some who were religious, but their expectation was of a false messiah of one sort or another. I hadn't yet learned that Jesus would be back quickly (Revelation 22:20).

Focusing on both wings of the New Age movement - the **occult exploration** of Satan's mysteries in the creation and the **protection** of that creation - I was missing the Creator. I didn't know that man had been created in order to have fellowship with the Creator. I didn't know that was what the Bible said. Mine was a New Age that *man* would build.

Unlike many New Agers, who unashamedly acknowledge the headship of Satan, I didn't think in terms of Satan either. I had learned 'healing' from a man who has been described as probably the most gifted psychic in the western world. I had prayed to an Indian 'god' and knew of his healing miracles. Many regard him as the most powerful psychic in the whole world. I had been 'healed' myself by a spiritual healer. However, by God's grace I was saved. My free will could never be taken from me. I asked Jesus into my life and by the miracle of being born again I came into the new life found in Jesus.

Whilst many New Agers are awaiting a one-world leader according to their faith or tradition, as a Bible-believing Christian I was soon to see what God says in His word. The part of my testimony that follows doesn't relate directly to healing or alternative medicine. However it is included to put into a wider context what *Christians* are discerning in alternative medicine. *The world* will see the growth in alternative healing methods more and more in the context of the New Age. *Christians* will begin to see it more and more in the context of Bible prophecy.

> *For there shall arise false Christs, and false prophets, and shall shew great signs and wonders; insomuch that, if it were possible, they shall deceive the very elect* (Matthew 24:24).

> *But of that day and hour knoweth no man, no, not the angels of heaven, but my Father only.*
> *But as the days of Noe were, so shall also the coming of the Son of man be.*
> *For as in the days that were before the flood they were eating and drinking, marrying and giving in marriage, until the day that Noe entered the ark.*
> *And knew not until the flood came, and took them all away; so shall also the coming of the Son of man be...*
> *Watch therefore: for ye know not what hour your Lord doth come...*
> *Therefore be ye also ready: for in such an hour as ye think not the Son of man cometh* (Matthew 24: 36-44).

We do not know the day or the hour. We *do* know the bridegroom is preparing the bride.

Neither do we know the day or the hour of the world ruler and false prophet of Revelation 13. Yet surely Satan is already preparing the world to receive him. Christians and non-Christians alike are being deceived by Satan's wiles, perhaps as never before, as the bride is made ready.

I was always a peaceful sort of person. The New Agers are peaceful people. They identify with the occult, which is powerful, and not with materialism and politics. They have a remarkable unity, powerfully supported by the god of this world. The Bible says the earth's inhabitants will be called upon to worship the one world ruler

(Revelation 13: 12) and the New Age counterfeit bride is being made ready.

What further evidence is there that the time of the one world ruler may not be far off? The evidence for the end of the end times can be seen in many Scriptures. However, I continue my own testimony and, I trust, throw further light on developments in the New Age. Satan is busy in everything that is 'New Age.'

Commerce, finance, 666 and the end-times

Up to the time of searching in the occult realm, I was a businessman. I studied economics and government at university, and most of my working life had been spent in senior positions in commerce and finance, mainly with large international corporations.

Until I knew Jesus Christ I didn't have any *clear* understanding of inflation and the money system. I didn't understand the nature of inflation. I didn't know the dollar was weak. I didn't know that borrowing and overspending had galloped to such an extent that the dollar was bound to collapse. The Lord took me to this understanding by way of His word in Revelation 13: 16-18. *'And he causeth all, both small and great, rich and poor, free and bond, to receive a mark in their right hand, or in their foreheads:*

And that no man might buy and sell, save that he had the mark, or the name of the beast, or the number of his name.

Here is wisdom. Let him that hath understanding count the number of the beast: for it is the number of a man; and his number is six hundred threescore and six.'

The Bible spoke to me in Revelation 13 about the world ruler and the false prophet who forced everyone to receive a mark on his right hand or on his forehead. Without this they were unable to buy or sell. We are told that with insight and wisdom we can calculate the number of this beast, and the Bible actually gives the number; it is 666. Then I read in Revelation 14 of the description of the eternal destination for those that take the mark and worship the world ruler (the beast).

I studied the coding system★ we see on our groceries. I could see that 666 always appears in the bar coding. I could understand how the debit card would come in and replace the credit card, and I could see that 666 was in evidence on some cards as well. The computers were now so advanced that all banking could be with a card, without cheques or cash. I found this was already happening in various trial locations. It seemed logical, at least, that when the world's money system did collapse, as it would through the collapse of the dollar, this would be a time to bring in the 'cashless society' or card system. The security risks of the card system are formidable and have already been reckoned; there already exists the technology and equipment invisibly to mark the card detail in the forehead and the right hand. As I write this, there has just come to hand the details of a Christian Newsletter from California. I read that 6,000 in Sweden in a practical experiment, involving real buying and selling, have taken a mark. The mark is registered in a computer. It is a mark for life, it was painless, it was put on by a 'ray gun', and it will register in banks or wherever those marked decide to shop. The shopkeeper, we are told, simply runs an electronic pen over the mark and it instantly sends the customer's number to a computer centre from where all information of their transactions is sent to their bank. No money needs to be touched.

Subsequently it was confirmed that the mark was on the right hand, and the location for the experiment was the south-eastern part of Sweden. It was learned in

★ see *The New Money System* by Mary Stewart Relfe, PO Box 4038, Montgomery, Alabama 36104, USA (1983)

Sweden that similar experiments were being carried out in Japan and in one Latin American country. Also in Sweden, one senior bank official made a remark that seems significant. He thought the public weren't quite ready for the system yet but that the government might make it mandatory in two years.

We live in a world that has now gone far along the road of deception. Satan has blinded and made ears deaf. *'If any man have an ear, let him hear. He that leadeth into captivity shall go into captivity: he that killeth with the sword must be killed with the sword. Here is the patience and the faith of the saints.* (Revelation 13: 9-10) My prayer is that Christians make ready for the bridegroom and at the same time be alert to the enemy's devices in the New Age. Christians can see that the world is deceived. When we meditate on God's word, we can see that prophecy is being fulfilled. God is always faithful to His word, and what is written *must* come to pass.

14
'Healing' and cancer 'help' centres

The New Age is seeing the *organisation* of alternative medicine. We see the growing interest in the apostate churches. We see its infiltration into churches that Satan is bringing into that state. We see the opening of more 'Healing Centres' of every kind. As with the 'alternative medicines' themselves, the variety of establishment is seemingly endless. They can be headed up by people who would (quite fairly) describe themselves as 'leading psychics' with 'specialist' establishments. Others, more subtly, can be offering therapies which, away from the occult would be valuable. Often today they are super-smart and sophisticated. Whatever its image there may well be a variety of therapies on offer. It could be mainly a healing centre, beauty parlour, health food store or whatever. Therapies on offer alongside the 'cosmetic camouflage', the 'beauty therapy' and the 'simple food bar' will in these days include acupuncture, reflexology, relaxation, yoga and all the rest! The centres vary and yet they are the same! Small town establishments are springing up. Large retail chains now specialise in health foods with homoeopathic remedies, self-hypnotism cassette tapes, books on 'healing' and so on.

Satan will invariably latch on to what is good; he often starts with a Bible truth. He may start with the leaves that are for healing according to Ezekiel 47:12 and bring magic to bear upon them. He seeks to get us off balance.

'Focus on Jesus' becomes 'I don't exist'. We are always to focus on Jesus, but also to remember that Satan is the ruler of the world according to Scripture. He can masquerade as an angel of light, and although Jesus has won the victory on the cross, we are commissioned to battle in His name against the principalities and powers that are at work. There is much that is good in a Health Store. However, discerning Christians will beware the mixture that is to be found there in these days.

The occult is all from the same promoter and, however high-flown the motive, it is misguided. One cancer help centre in Britain is now known world-wide, after a very short time, and it is alarming to look at the lines of treatment available there:-

'Spiritual Healing', 'Faith Healing' or 'Magnetic Healing' is available from a 'Healer'. Self healing is a description given to another line of treatment there using breathing, relaxation, meditation of several types, bio-feedback and imaging on Simonton lines. After self healing there is 'self enquiry' where the idea is to look into one's psychology aided by counsellors teaching several methods including Jungian, psycho-synthesis, hypnosis, etc. according to what seem to be individual needs. Also there are Bach remedies supposed to balance emotional deficiencies. They encourage other therapies such as acupuncture, herbalism and homoeopathy.

Another line of treatment is the metabolic regime which consists mainly of vitamins (some in large doses), minerals, enzymes, and immune stimulation and support. Diet is important and another line of treatment includes a three-month cleansing period. There is a raw vegetable, fruit and grain diet with little fat, no salt, no refined carbohydrates, no sugar, coffee or milk. After that people who need meat can go on to small amounts of fish, chicken and eggs.

The establishment of this centre is an extraordinary milestone in the progress of 'alternative medicine'. The lines of treatment outlined above represent a typical package found in this sort of establishment, and it is understood that they intend to expand the number of therapies. This range, and the support received from so many places, is a measure of the longing on everybody's part to find some right answers to the dreadful health problem of our age — cancer. Indeed the centre has responded to a spiritual need. Whilst its critics have majored on the lack of science, the problem is indeed in the dimension the centre has brought into focus. Also nothing should be taken away from the sincerity, commitment, care and willingness to help that lies behind the motives of this sort of centre. My plea is for discernment.

The purpose of this book is to caution that there are two realms in the spiritual dimension, and to encourage Christians mindful of their responsibility (1 Cor. 2:14) to seek the discernment to know if a particular therapy is of God.

I believe I have made it clear that spiritual therapies which are not of God are very dangerous. Commitment, care and sincerity on the part of the unknowing helpers, understandably eager to support their fellow men in the times of their greatest need, serves only to promote the activity of deceiving spirits.

The following is the testimony of a born again believer who visited the centre I have mentioned:

'In August of last year I had a mastectomy. A few weeks previously I had seen a programme about a cancer clinic. It interested me because people seemed caring, and were seeking to help and support people who had had cancer or were facing it long term.

'In hospital a young woman with a few weeks to live was seeking the Lord. She had been to the clinic and wondered if it could meet her need. I promised her I would go and see. It proved to be very traumatic.

'Making an early start, I was taken by a friend whose

husband had died of cancer. We were met at the door by a sincere, very nice, caring person, but as I went into the clinic a feeling of oppression seemed to meet me. The first person I saw asked where the cancer was. They raised their hands above me. I asked if they prayed, and was told they did not. Feeling the power of the enemy, I asked the Lord for the protection of the precious blood. I felt very vulnerable because I was so low physically, spiritually, emotionally and in every way.

'Each person that dealt with me was caring, the message coming through that if one had peace it was possible to beat or help the cancer. In the meditation session I again felt the need of the protection of the precious blood, a feeling that grew throughout the day.

'Diet was discussed. A lot of what they said was sincere, caring, and supportive to the patients. The friends and relations had sessions too. The friend that took me had the same feeling about the place.

'I had not realised before going that it was spirit healing, not Christian healing from the Lord. The spiritist healing was not really evident until one got there and read the literature that was left around for folk to read. I came back feeling it would be so important to have a Christian based clinic.'

Sally, who wrote that testimony, is, on any view, a mature born again believer with a lifetime of mission behind her. So often the error is not obvious until we look closer; Sally **visited** the centre. I have been to it too, and have been well received there. My prayer, along with a group of other Christians, has been that the place will become Christ-centred, and, failing that, that it will be closed. However the centre expands, and more centres are opening, and are well supported by influential people. The range of therapies is large. Many more therapists are being trained in these days, and it is understandable that centres open to accommodate them. In the town nearest to my home, the healing centre presents an attractive image. It seems set to grow in popularity and perhaps challenge the practitioners of medical science.

The Bible foretells the signs of the end of the age. *'Watch out no-one deceives you'*. When we get man's natural initiative and drive behind the promotion of these therapies and centres, the deception will be formidable. Many are living in fear of cancer. Particularly in the United States, the statistics show a large growth in this disease. The Imperial Cancer Research Fund tells us, 'In England and Wales, one person in four is likely to develop cancer at some time in their life and one in five will die of it.' However the truth is in God's word, **not** in forecasted statistics.

The method of one New Age 'searcher' group aims to eliminate the destructive elements in the existing system of treatment so that the new holistic approach is complementary to it; also it is directed towards setting right the destructive elements within the individual which are believed to have contributed to the development of the cancer. The patient is encouraged to believe that he himself can control or even destroy the cancer, through correcting what are called the forces of personality and emotion, through counselling, psychotherapy, deep relaxation, meditation and creative visualisation. This recognises that cancer is a disease of the total system and that tumours are but an indicator of these disorders.

What we need to recognise is that Satan can not only produce the cancer but that some of these cancer treatments are from Satan too. We need to be aware that there are sincere and well-intentioned groups, displaying impressive medical credentials and the language of a false spirituality, who are tapping into the wrong spiritual realm, without knowledge of Jesus, and without regard for His word.

15
Churches off the track

As well as looking critically at the 'alternative medicines' and so-called healing establishments, Christians do well from the healing point-of-view to look closely at the denominational churches. Look also at the agencies they proliferate as they move into the spiritual dimension, often with no clear view of the two realms that are to be found there.

Consider for example the Churches' Fellowship for Psychical and Spiritual Studies. The name describes the purpose of the fellowship. Do they forget that dabbling, even for the seeker after a new psychical and biblical approach to psychical or spiritual phenomena is forbidden by God and invokes Satan's spell? In a Quarterly Review in 1982 we could read that 'mediumship is a potential gift of the Holy Spirit'.

A national Anglican journal on healing recently featured the healing practised by the Healer whose radio programme started me off on the 'search'. Before that search eventually led me to Jesus I had attended his training centre and he had been one of my teachers.

Scripture allows no grey area between God and Satan. My own passage from darkness into light was a remarkable miracle. I had met with many caring and sincere teachers and I had witnessed their power to 'heal'. I do not know how to explain what it means to be a new creation to those who are working counterfeit miracles. I do not know how to explain it to many in the churches.

It is clear we have many apostate churches which have

departed so far from the truth that unity with them is impossible.

Recently I attended evensong at a major Anglican church. The proposed extension of its healing ministry was described on the notice board outside, but to enter I had to pass through a T'ai Chi class in progress in the church hallway.

Beware also books on spiritual subjects, which have only a *superficial* Christian appearance. In books brought to the discerning it can soon become clear where there is error. A foreword by a former bishop for example, provided no clue to the status of the healing sanctuary the author (himself a clergyman) had set out to describe. Another foreword by a different former bishop once again gave a credibility to what was therein discussed. The subject was acupuncture!

God is no respecter of persons; we are all equal before Him. We do well as Christians to test all ideas for error. Without discernment this is so easily mixed with truth.

At one conference I was shown for the first time a book for which the Holy Spirit had prepared me some months previously. It was just one of many books of New Age teaching on healing from professing Christian authors today. The publishers had described it as controversial, but such a book needed discernment more than discussion. The cover described the author's amazing gift and how he discovered a remarkable new method of healing. A book from the occult (which I had burned when I came to know Jesus) was referred to in it and a quick follow-through showed no hint of disapproval by the author. Progress through the book provided confirmation upon confirmation of the initial discernment.

I believe the Lord taught me a lesson through this book. It was clear to me the book wasn't Holy Spirit led and I marked line after line that jarred with my spirit. Then one day I was asked by two mature Christians, one a general medical practitioner, to go through the book with them to explain my objections. For two hours I attempted to do that. I failed. I couldn't convey what the Holy Spirit was so clearly saying, and about halfway through the book the three of us gave up. I hadn't convinced them on a single point. 'But we can see you are right about the book,' they told me afterwards. The Lord had given them discernment too. This book is a plea for the exercise of spiritual discernment. We can only receive it from Him. Some have written to me evidencing that same discernment; on the other hand it seems a great number of Christians remain deceived. One review described it as an important book and then went on to reproduce its errors. Then I was greatly encouraged to read in a later issue of the same publication, a warning by the editor to readers about the book. He quoted an Australian authority who has recognised much of the teaching of this book to be similar to that of the Spiritualist Church, and rooted in the occult. I believe more Christians must speak out and admonish with all wisdom (Colossians 3:16). Often it seems there are but a few who spot deceptions, and when they do, so often it seems they do not speak out.

I have related those areas that I believe God has specifically brought to my attention. Nearer to where I live, I have twice visited one particular church. Each occasion was for the visit of a psychic 'healer'. Once I was a 'searcher' in Satan's kingdom, and once a member of the Church.

Beware therefore those places and those leaders who once brought glory to God but where in these days Satan appears to be dimming the light. Prayer is needed for the *real* leaders in our established church for they have many in their ranks who, far from having discernment, do not even believe that Jesus Christ is the Son of God. And yet they may have a ministry for 'healing'!

We can no longer afford to ignore the spiritual status of those that minister healing to us - that goes for the

181

churches as well as for the whole field of medicine.

Visiting a cancer help centre in 1983, I had seen the occult with a *medical* label; I saw occult therapies gaining more respectability. In 1984, I hoped I would not see a parallel situation, with a *Christian* label, when I made a special journey to London to attend the monthly healing service at the church I mentioned earlier, a place I believe God had put on my heart since stumbling into the T'ai Chi class being held in the church the year before. On my journey I was able to read a magazine devoted to healing, and connected with this church. The magazine, still asking the wrong dangerous questions, 'Does Alternative Therapy Work?' in its front page headline, set out the 'Order of Service' I would be attending that evening.

I was conscious of the need for unity. However I had read what David Watson had written★ about the two main dangers for believers: "One is unity where there ought to be division, the other is division where there ought to be unity ... But there can be no true unity where there are basic differences over essentials of the faith, such as the deity of Christ, the atonement, justification by faith, the resurrection of Christ, the necessity of new birth or the authority of scripture." I had fasted. I had time to pray, and I didn't know if I could be in unity with them.

A copy of an article in the London *Standard* (February 1983) on the board outside the church gave much information about the conversion of the crypt into a healing centre. There was a photograph of Princess Caroline of Monaco and the new foundation stone commemorating her visit; work on the healing centre had begun. Also on the board was a letter from the World Health Organisation in Geneva. This serves very well to

★ *Hidden Warfare* by David Watson (STL Books - 1972)

emphasise the significance of the centre on the world scene, and the interest of the World Health Organisation should not be regarded as insignificant! The letter included the following:

It seems certain that this Centre, serving those in need of affirmation and wholeness will become a pattern for future developments in health care. As the industrialised societies become progressively more complex and bewildering, the need becomes ever more apparent, and specific action to meet it becomes an urgent demand.
We will be watching the progress of the Centre with great interest and commend it to the generosity of those you approach.

The burden of Christians has to be that the Centre, when opened, will be Christ centred; the leadership at the centre will need to turn to scripture to find the path it has to travel.

The Churches' Council for Health and Healing (CCHH) seeks to help and encourage the churches. It produces a directory, *Your Very Good Health* which lists many health and healing organisations. The Council was set up 40 years ago by Archbishop William Temple; but it seems the scene now is a very different one. Striking advances have been made into occult medicine and we have to look at the CCHH as it is today.

They see the person as a whole - body, mind and spirit - in intimate and dynamic interaction. However they seem to miss some vital scriptures. *Your Very Good Health* includes groups because of the 'quality' of their work, and it describes one organisation which has the main aim of developing 'all forms of yoga.' The aim of another is to secure the passing of laws to recognise 'natural healers.' 'Health in the New Age' is another group listed. This aims to be a **bridge** between scientists,

183

doctors, ministers of religion and practitioners of alternative medicine on the one side, and lay men on the other. At the time of the directory listing, the same charitable trust was described as advising the 'Festival of Mind, Body and Spirit'. The trust was actively promising the idea of an international association for 'Holistic Health Care' to work officially with the World Health Organisation. Also it was setting up a 'New Age Information Service' to link via computer to organisations in Europe and the United States.

Christians led by the Holy Spirit work better than synods, councils and bureaucracies. It is the same with these New Age 'networks'. They work well. One organisation listed is the 'Positive Health Network', established to develop 'wide' contacts in the area of health. Yet another organisation stated its aim as teaching the diagnosis and correction of energy imbalances. Another trust listed — well known to those of us who have moved in the occult realm — is described as helping 'seekers' to find the discipline that suits *them* best.

Throughout the Directory, I see little evidence of what *God* wants. Rather we are presented with an assortment including a great deal that is occult. There is the implicit invitation to see what suits *us* best. Indeed there is a marked absence of scripture. In the lengthy introduction, the General Secretary of the CCHH says he has 'no doubt' that the contributions of the 'ecological field', the 'personal growth movement' and the recovery of a spiritual dimension through yoga or zen, or by a return to a religious way of seeing reality, are all vital. Away from the evils evidenced in pills and depressions, the General Secretary looks optimistically to communities being 'inventive' including food habits and 'spiritual healing'.

As I read the directory I was reminded of my weekend at a retreat. I had just heard of the discovery of my fellow searcher's naked and mutilated body. My friend was dead with wounds self inflicted through demonic influences and I had, as a consequence, started to search into the dangers of my search and my discoveries. At that retreat I was able to buy another directory of the occult. Also on the notice boards I was confronted with posters and advertising of the sort I was by this time trying to escape. I remember thinking my search into the occult, then ending, could have progressed much faster, had I visited this place at the outset. The same would be true with the wealth of information the CCHH provided.

Let us also beware of counterfeit gifts even in fellowships of committed Christians. **Occult laying-on-of-hands** exists where we least expect to find it! Satan seeks to pervert the true healing in the name of Jesus. He will encourage sincere ritual healing, spoken in the name of Jesus by those who don't know Him and where it can't be truly in Jesus' name at all.

As we have seen, in Matthew 7: 21-23 Jesus is reminding us that we have to *know* Him. We must have the Holy Spirit dwelling in us if we are to do the Father's will. We need to watch out for false prophets who find platforms in Christian fellowships. We need to beware too of those ministers who, without discernment, encourage all and sundry to lay hands on other members of a congregation. In this supernatural dimension, Satan, the deceiver, awaits his opportunity; he knows the supernatural better than the finest Christian minister who will be helpless without discernment. *'But I fear, lest by any means, as the serpent beguiled Eve through his subtilty, so your minds should be corrupted from the simplicity that is in Christ'* (2 Cor 11:3). The truth is found in God's word. Alternative medicine is in large part a counterfeit of divine healing; false prophets on the Christian circuit can present an even more subtle challenge. Discernment is essential.

New Age Healing Deceptions in the Church

Since the Second Edition of this book was written it has been plain to many that deceptions of various kinds in the area of healing are to be found in the Church and throughout the body of true believers. What we are seeing is a focus apart from the Lord, another man-pleasing gospel. This has resulted in a new language being spoken and the messages of Positive Confession, of 'Power Evangelism' and Signs and Wonders, of Inner Healing and of Psychology are being heard more and more widely through conferences, videos, audio message tapes and all the rest. These messages serve as a channel for methods belonging to the New Age and the occult and which have no place in Christian life. They are akin to the so-called holistic health care methods of Alternative Medicine; there is much New Age teaching in the Church in these days.

'Signs and Wonders' ★

It is a real danger in teaching 'signs and wonders' that whilst the teaching may be good, the class or congregation, big or small, with new or with mature believers, may be unable to receive it. Others may not even *know* Jesus. Surely there are leaders and teachers who do not recognise those who don't *know* Jesus; the job is made more difficult by what is really a new 'form of godliness'. This can take the form of impressive 'praise and worship', tongues and manifestation of various 'gifts' by those who simply have no fruits. It is by their

★ First appeared in *Understanding Deception - New Age Teaching in the Church* (New Wine Press - 1987)

fruits we shall know them. Do they even *know* Jesus? There is a real need for discernment.

The teaching materials of the one 'Signs and Wonders' teacher I believe God has constantly brought to my attention show a lack of discernment. Many who *do* know very well that demons *can* counterfeit physical healing (even though they put something much worse than the original sickness in its place) often have little discernment when demonic activity comes into a *Christian* fellowship. Discernment is greatly needed in the body of Christ in these days when the Holy Spirit is at work.

Occult activity is increasing too; it surely must according to Scripture and if it is to sustain Antichrist who will come in the flesh. Teaching that encourages signs and wonders *must* include more than a passing reference to discernment.

Psychology★

While psycholgists are passing on from their Man-centred studies into spiritual transpersonal psychology, Christians are getting sucked into the psychology system at the other end of the pipe line. These Christians, many of them already experiencing supernatural power in their ministries, must beware of the traps that can await even those who who venture a single step into this most subtle deception. The way Man behaves if he doesn't walk with God is very different from the way when he does! Psychology and Christianity have little in common. They both seek to explain Man's behaviour but each has its own solution, and our caution against the methods of

★ First appeared in *Understanding Deception - New Age Teaching in the Church* (New Wine Press - 1987)

psychology is not any denial of the essential human element in Man.

Visiting America after renouncing Moral Re-Armament (MRA) as a cult I asked Robert Vlerick, a teacher of Spiritual Warfare, the one who first identified the New Age Movement to me, if he knew any cult that was more subtle than MRA. His answer was immediate and without qualification: psychology. If the Bible is true then psychology only offers what we do not need. Psychology pretends to scientifically understand the heart of man, and so denies our spiritual nature and our free will. Psychology encourages us to improve ourselves rather than to submit ourselves broken and fit to be used by the living God. One doesn't have to be a Christian to know that pride abounds throughout the human race, but today according to much of the teaching the problem is supposed to lie in our **lack of self worth** or our **humility.**

Christians getting involved with the methods of psychology such as we shall see with Inner Healing need to understand that they are getting involved with a focus on self, and it is but a step further when they are led into the area known as transpersonal psychology, the spiritual way more akin to the magical ways of the eastern religions.

Visualisation and Inner Healing ★

If there is one area that is very significant in the end-time deception, and yet which Christians are finding so difficult to understand, it is visualisation. I urge Christians to ask the Lord for this understanding. We

★ First appeared in *Understanding Deception - New Age Teaching in the Church* (New Wine Press - 1987)

wrestle against the authorities, against the powers of this dark world and against the spiritual forces of evil in the heavenly realm (Ephesians 6:12).

Visualisation is a very basic tool of operation in the occult realm and it has its foot very well into the Christian door. We have considered the subject previously but it is necessary to introduce it again here. It is a major technique of Inner Healing. It is valuable to look at visualisation again.

Inner Healing is just one — a most significant one — of the many therapies taken on by believers and Christianised by them as they came into the charismatic 'renewal' wanting to 'move with the spirit' and bring wholeness, such as *they* had received to *others*. Unfortunately they have set up ministries based upon psychology. That's all very well up to a point. Psychology has given us a clearer understanding of the unredeemed human character, but it fails to give biblical answers.

I do not pretend to bring any experience in Christian counselling, and I hesitate to come forward with easy alternatives to the visualisation methods of Inner Healing that are so unacceptable. There *are* great things to be achieved through good *scripturally-sound* counselling for the emotional areas. However I believe there are three things that are worth remembering in the context of our analysis here:

Firstly, we all have to grow as Christians and the process of renewing the mind continues only as the subject wills. Also it takes time.

Secondly, with our will again, we can determine to do what has to be done. If we have received God's forgiveness and love, how can we withhold it from our earthly father, our grandfather, our grandmother, and all the rest that today's Inner Healers almost inevitably come up with as keys to a seemingly difficult situation? We have to make a choice to forgive. The Inner Healer, though sincerely trying hard and believing himself to be hearing God, is almost invariably in the driving seat himself. For myself, one who has enjoyed good parental care and a very happy childhood, I also find difficulty in accepting the comparison of the earthly father to the heavenly Father in the way that the Inner Healers commonly do. Our heavenly God is far beyond such earthly comparison.

Thirdly, we can petition God; we can pray.

Prayer is the way through and God does meet the needs of the emotionally hurt. Counselling should help towards this goal, enabling the person in need to make the choice to forgive.

Satan has more than one way to promote the ultimate lie that we can be like God and many in the churches have unknowingly come to believe it. Our walk with the Lord as believers is a walk of faith. Believing is not the same thing as imagining or visualising, which are neither taught nor encouraged anywhere in Scripture. However visualisation is well understood by those familiar with the occult realm. It is a most powerful way of tuning in to the spirit world.

When we speak of visualising and imagining it must of course be acknowledged that there are non-occult senses of these words. I believe it will be clear that what I write is not referring to these, nor is it referring to what the Lord can sovereignly do. Our reference is to Man's methods of influencing reality. It is one thing to visualise the sort of house we ask an architect to design or the garden we are planning. It is quite another to visualise all the seats in a church to be full when they are empty, or little men with hammers within the body attacking cancer cells. The ends may be in God's will, but the methods have to be His also. These are both real examples from my experience. If it suits his purpose Satan can bring a counterfeit healing but in any event our departure into fantasy (a misplaced faith) gives demons both the invitation and the opportunity.

And God saw that the wickedness of man was great in the earth, and that every imagination of the thoughts of his heart was only evil continually (Genesis 6:5).

The truth of this scripture can be hard for many Christians to receive. Imagination and fantasy may well *seem* harmless enough, yet the Bible describes them as evil. Those who have had experience in witchcraft do not have the same difficulty. It has to be emphasised: visualisation is very dangerous.

Once again Hunt and McMahon's 'The Seduction of Christianity' is an invaluable reference book for those who need to see how visualisation has become such a significant tool, and how it has come through from the occultists and so-called 'thinkers' of the past to believers who are at the front in some of the 'signs and wonders' ministries seen today. The report of one institute states that the use of the imagination is one of the most rapidly spreading new trends in psychology and education.

Materialisation also is known in the occult realm and psychologists today are well into this sort of deception too. As one psychologist put it, if when we eat an apple and it becomes energy, or mind, it should not be difficult to grasp that the *thought* (or imagination) of an apple is capable of becoming an apple again - not an imagined apple but a real one. When we start to put faith in our imaginations, we are starting on a very slippery slope.

Jung was an occult psychiatrist and according to one teacher at the C G Jung Institute in the United States, visualisation or imagery is considered the most powerful tool in Jungian psychology for achieving direct contact with the unconscious and attaining 'greater inner knowledge.' This transpersonal psychology is the psychology of 'transcendent experience' and it is at this level of psychology that East meets West.

This transcendentalism gave rise to the 'New Thought' which we see in the idea that 'thought', or the mind, controls all things. We see in the secular world the growth of interest in 'Mind over Matter' pursuits such as karate and judo. Parallel with this New Age activity, there is inside the church a spirit tempting with the idea that God is not personal but a great *Mind* that can be activated through our own *minds*. The only answer is Jesus.

Positive confession

To have true faith is to trust God that He will do what He has said He will do in His word.

All of Satan's deceptions are based upon a truth and there is of course *some* truth in the teaching of the 'Faith' people because we are told to walk by faith. It is a basic requirement of the Christian walk.

However the 'Faith' or 'Positive Confession' movement is taking Christians to the line that has to be drawn between Holy Spirit ministries and sorcery. It is when we neglect the importance of receiving truth from the Word through the revelation of the Holy Spirit, often due to a concentration on the positive that we *believe* God wants for us, that sorcery is not far away.

The truth or the positive? ★

When we leave the truth to concentrate on 'positive' goals sorcery is not far away.

In 'Beyond Seduction' ★★ Dave Hunt writes, "what actually matters is not whether something is 'positive' but whether something is true or false, biblical or not

★ First appeared in *Understanding Deception - New Age Teaching in the Church* (New Wine Press - 1987)

★★ Published by Harvest House, Eugene, Oregon - 1987

biblical. In that context, then, the terms 'positive' or 'negative' are not only irrelevant but a smokescreen that obscures real issues.'' Referring to the '*strong delusion*' to believe Satan's lie (2 Thessalonians 2: 9-12) about which Paul warned those who were not lovers of the truth, Hunt continues: ''The popular substitution of 'positive' for 'truth' is a perfect set-up for the prophesied delusion.''

Isn't it perfectly clear that the Bible, positive for the gospel it contains, is cram full of negatives which men ignore at their peril? Isn't it certain that Genesis 2:17 contains a vital *negative*? It reads:

> *But of the tree of the knowledge of good and evil, thou shalt not eat of it: for in the day that thou eatest thereof thou shalt surely die.*

There is a clear line to be drawn between Holy Spirit ministries and sorcery. The experience from America shows that not only are Christian ministries very close to or over that line but also that they are hardly distinguishable from those which have never been on the Christian side. Napoleon Hill is one who has a following among Christians and, as Hunt and McMahon point out, ★ it is interesting that Christians recommending his writings (his famous title is 'Think and Grow Rich'), if offering any caution, do so as regards the *wealth* aspect. The dangers of the mind power involved pass undiscerned. Peace of mind can be dangerous when it is counterfeit; my own embarkation into the occult began with counterfeit peace of mind. In his book, 'Grow Rich with Peace of Mind' Napoleon Hill describes the 'unseen friends' that sometimes 'hover' about him. He has discovered

---

★ *The Seduction of Christianity* by Dave Hunt (Harvest House, Eugene, Oregon - 1985)

there is a group of strange beings who maintain a school of wisdom with 'Masters' who can disembody themselves and travel instantly to wherever they choose. Sadly Napoleon Hill is tapped into the occult realm.

Hill's 'Positive Mental Attitudes' are close to those of another group, the 'Positive Possibility Thinkers'. Dave Hunt tells us that these have their roots in 'New Thought', a group which emphasised that thought controlled everything. "The power of thinking, whether negative or positive, was believed to be sufficient even to create physical reality or to destroy it. God was not personal, but a Great Mind which was activated by our thoughts and would actualise them into concrete form. The corollary of this axiom is obvious: Man is divine." ★ He tells us this was once forced out of the church as a heresy only to survive in cults like Christian Science. "Today's church is being swept by a revival of New Thought, now called Positive Thinking, Positive Confession, Positive Mental Attitude, and Inner Healing. We are very concerned that this time New Thought, which represents inside the church what New Age is in the secular world, will not be forced out, but will remain within the Evangelical Church to contribute to the growing confusion and seduction. One of the most basic New Thought techniques is visualisation, which is now firmly entrenched within the church." ★

The great need is for discernment in the body of believers. I believe the Lord has that Gift of Discernment of Spirits for us (1 Corinthians 12:10) and also He has given us His Word; as Christians, we have to check out the teaching we receive from men to see whether it is written there (Acts 17:11).

★ *The Seduction of Christianity* by Dave Hunt (Harvest House, Eugene, Oregon - 1985)

16
The healing network

Alternative medicine, including the most devastatingly dangerous psychic and spiritual healing therapies, is fast growing in acceptability. It is getting itself highly organised too. We see associations and alliances that are bringing together out-and-out spiritualists with nominal, and even born again, Christians. The Confederation of Healing Organisations (CHO) was founded in 1981 and comprises nine organisations. The National Federation of Spiritual Healers, the well known established organisation for spiritual healers, all their spiritualist associations, and the Radionic Association, are included. The Churches' Council for Health and Healing is given 'observer' status. The CHO cooperates with the Natural Health Network. Recently this body brought together delegates from all over Britain to listen to speakers on the theme 'Natural Health and its Place in Society.'

Apart from the precedents being set by the Healing Centres and some 'Christian' churches in the same period we have seen medical doctors form the British Holistic Medical Association. We have seen the formation of the British Holistic Pharmacists Association. Still in the same short period, the monthly *Journal of Alternative Medicine* provided excellent PR for alternative medicine. For the layman we have seen the launch of an attractive magazine *Alternative Medicine Today* which focused on Prince Charles' views in its first issue. We have seen vast numbers of new books about alternative therapies. We have witnessed the support of nominally Christian churches for all that is taking place.

Prince Charles attended a colloquium on the subject organised by the Royal Society of Medicine, and the 'Journal of Alternative Medicine' reported (September 1984) that under Sir James Watt, Past President of the Society, it is beginning to take a leading role in offering suggestions for integrating complimentary and allopathic medicine.

The representative of the British Holistic Medical Association opened the colloquium and (according to the Journal) the central issue between allopathic and alternative medicine was seen like this:

> It would seem that the energetic or vitalistic principles which describe the body's homeostasis in many of the alternative therapies do have a sound basis in theoretical physics and chemistry. These concepts have been largely ignored by the majority of 'scientific and academic' doctors, who instead have concentrated on material phenomena, some of which are of questionable scientific value.

That seems to be a fair summary of the position between alternative and allopathic medicine as the majority of their respective practitioners see it. Also we can look at it in this way:

1. Doctors, guided as far as possible by science and intelligent observations on a 'Does it work?' basis, have indeed concentrated on material aspects.

2. These same scientifically minded doctors have hitherto, and in spite of their own use of placebo treatments, failed to see that the alternative treatments (cloaked in the deceptive ideas about energy) *do* work. At the very least they can work when faith is put in them.

Admittedly the Royal Society of Medicine has laid down criteria for collaboration, namely a recognised training programme, recognised qualifications, a self-regulatory organisation and a willingness to submit their results to research. That will naturally exclude many of the fringe alternative therapies not seen as providing a satisfactory basis for collaboration with the medical profession. Nevertheless the criteria will encourage many of the therapies and the gates will be opened to them. Next we can expect that the practitioners of the less significant therapies will not be slow in putting their houses in acceptable administrative order to get the same recognition.

For those who meet the criteria, the Royal Society of Medicine has been at great pains to avoid the term 'alternative'. They say this suggests competition between orthodox and other therapies, and they prefer the term 'complementary'.

The effect of such dialogues involving distinguished, and even learned, participants is to lend weight to the idea that alternative medicine is scientific. Additionally there is the pressure of the increasing evidence, now coming through to the general public, that orthodox medicine is not as scientific as had been supposed. Too long the medical doctors have prescribed on the basis of 'Does it work?' without knowing some of the hidden dangers; now they are being forced to look at what seem to be some very attractive alternatives. These *do* work, and it is likely they will work even 'better' given the psychology of a medical doctor's prescription and endorsement. Doctors are being led from the fairly obvious dangers that accompany many of the existing conventional treatments, into the subtle and seemingly danger-free world of the 'natural' therapies.

This swing from drugs to the even more dangerous occult therapies is a parallel of the swing seen on the seedier side of the drug world. There we see movement on from the drug called cannabis or marijuana through a whole range and on to various forms of yoga and meditation. The prayers of Christians are urgently needed in this whole area (Ephesians 6: 18).

- And in the churches

Many believers remain in apostate churches and can therefore hardly escape the apostate teaching. How long dare they hang on? What example do they set the unsaved? How do they dare to bring others into fellowship there? How long can they remain there as the spiritual forces accelerate against them? How will they receive the miracles when they witness them, and how will they know if they are from Satan? Are they really strong enough to stand, even as missionaries, in a fellowship where Jesus is not Lord? Do they believe there can be fellowship when Christ is not at the centre of it? Indeed will our Lord allow unity where He is left out? Where can we find in Scripture any basis for being pastored by an unbeliever?

The Psalmist tells us, *'Blessed is the man that walketh not in the counsel of the ungodly'* (Psalm 1:1). Paul had this to say to the believers at Corinth:

Be ye not unequally yoked together with unbelievers: for what fellowship hath righteousness with unrighteousness? and what communion hath light with darkness?
And what concord hath Christ with Belial? or what part hath he that believeth with an infidel?
And what agreement hath the temple of God with idols? for ye are the temple of the living God; as God hath said, I will dwell in them, and walk in them; and I will be their God, and they shall be my people.

> *Wherefore come out from among them, and be ye*
> *separate, saith the Lord, and touch not the unclean*
> *thing; and I will receive you,*
> *And will be a Father unto you, and ye shall be my sons*
> *and daughters, saith the Lord Almighty,*
> (2 Corinthians 6: 14-18).

Ignoring Scripture will prove dangerous for believers who remain in apostate churches. Christians will need to beware when they start to see miracles at the hands of unbelievers. Jesus doesn't mind where His healing is manifested. However Satan will be especially pleased to 'heal' in the churches when the way is made open for him! Satan's healing network seems set for advances in that direction.

Those who continue to fellowship under the ministry of unbelievers will do so at their peril.

> *This know also, that in the last days perilous times*
> *shall come.*
> *For men shall be lovers of their own selves, covetous,*
> *boasters, proud, blasphemers, disobedient to parents,*
> *unthankful, unholy,*
> *Without natural affection, trucebreakers, false*
> *accusers, incontinent, fierce, despisers of those that*
> *are good,*
> *Traitors, heady, highminded, lovers of pleasures more*
> *than lovers of God;*
> *Having a form of godliness, but denying the power*
> *thereof: from such turn away* (2 Timothy 3: 1-5).

Thus Paul wrote of the circumstances in our own day, and of the *form* of godliness that we know so well today.

17
The World Health Organisation and The World Council of Churches

In July 1984 I travelled to Geneva to visit the World Health Organisation (WHO) and the Christian Medical Commission (CMC) which is part of the World Council of Churches (WCC). Living away from London I very rarely see the London *Standard*. The headline caught my eye on the news stand as I passed through the airport building: 'Charles, the would-be healer.' 'I've always wished that I could heal.' Inside I read, 'From exercise to extra-sensory perception, from coping with stress to self-discipline... the sincere and outspoken views of the Prince of Wales.' A special four-page pull-out centred on the interview given by the Prince to a reporter at Kensington Palace.

On my journey I could read how it was that Charles 'happened' to settle his eyes on a book about Paracelsus as he pondered what he would say in his speech to the British Medical Association (already referred to on page 27). I read how he believed it was only by being 'open' that we could encourage others to be the same. I recalled how 'open' I had been on the day my search into healing methods began when I just 'happened' to switch on BBC Radio at a very unusual time of the day and there 'happened' to be just starting a programme telling us of our potential as healers. Jesus was not then Lord of my life.

The next day in Geneva, the Manager of the Traditional Medicine Programme at the WHO was enthusiastically copying the words for the *Standard* we had open before us. Here was a Nigerian medical doctor, fairly recently appointed to this top job in this well respected United Nations agency. But what of the World Health Organisation itself? What of its traditional medicine programme? Traditional medicine is really another description for alternative medicine, and whatever the native names, I soon established that it was a case of 'the same mixture as before.' My host and I, there in his office, were surrounded with all the evidence of occult medicine including the life-sized acupuncture chart that dominated the wall behind him.

A book, ★ put together by his predecessor, 344 pages of the world's traditional medicine, seemed to confirm all the indications as to the direction the WHO is headed. In his foreword to the book, Halfdan Mahler, MD, tells us of its purpose in providing a better understanding of 'traditional, indigenous and unorthodox' systems. In what seemed a significant conclusion, he writes, 'It is hoped that this information will be of use to governments when they consider the most appropriate methods for inclusion in their health strategies.'

In these days we see governments taking a new look at their health plans and training programmes. The five-year plan for traditional medicine, upon which the WHO has recently embarked, seems set to bring about a new understanding and availability of the enormous choice that there is. There is no discernment; indeed this large

★ *Traditional Medicine and Health Care Coverage* (WHO - Geneva) - 1983

book has chapter upon chapter dealing with therapies clearly recognised by Christians as occult.

It is inevitably true that the basis of the medicine in the great majority of the WHO member countries is traditional rather than what we call scientific. However it is a significant sign of the times we are in, that traditional medicine was only incorporated into the WHO programmes as recently as 1976. In that same year the World Council of Churches shifted its perspective also. I believe the present programme is especially significant. In the jargon of the United Nations, this new 'Global Medium-term Programme 12.3 - Traditional Medicine' appears for the first time as part of 'Objective 12'. It involves the aim of fostering national and international action to achieve specified objectives by 1989. The first objective is for those countries where traditional medicine is widely practised; they are to have 'useful' traditional practices incorporated into their general system of health care. For the second objective, the WHO wants to identify at least two centres for research in traditional medicine in each region. The United Kingdom is one of the thirty-three active member states in the European Region. The Regional Office for Europe is in Copenhagen, Denmark but it would perhaps be surprising if there was not a Centre for research established in Britain. Also part of the plan is to identify as many 'traditional medicine plants or treatments' as possible.

Again predictably, 'Does it work?' is the question being asked. 'Does it come from the spiritual dimension, and if so, which realm?': that is the question to which science and Satan has blinded us.

One chapter of *Traditional Medicine and Health Care Coverage* is contributed by one of the leaders of the Holistic Health Movement from England. He deals with Anthroposophical Medicine, Autogenic Training, Bates Technique, Breathing, Biofeedback, Colour Therapy,

Flower Remedies, Gerson Treatment, Healing, Hydrotherapy, Negative Ions, Radionics, Reflexology (Zone Therapy), Shiatsu, Do-In and T'ai Chi.

Could there be a place in this traditional medicine programme at the WHO for Divine Healing? I recalled that the large and glossy alternative medicine books sometimes gave one page to this. Now that the WHO had come into the spiritual and supernatural dimension it occured to me there might be an openness to the idea of looking at Divine Healing. My reply came in a letter from the WHO: 'There are very firm guidelines laid down by the Organisation for its programme of traditional medicine and these preclude the possibility of integrating certain aspects of traditional medicine based on spiritual, moral or other fundamental principles.'

Only four hundred yards or so from the place of my meeting at the WHO, the Central Committee of the World Council of Churches was in session. It is undeniable that there are Christians at work in these organisations and condemnation is neither appropriate nor intended. However the likelihood of both of them having a significant part in the one-world government prophesied in the Book of Revelation must be worth mentioning. *'If any man have an ear, let him hear'* (Revelation 13: 9).

The Archbishop of York had left behind the problems of his office and I was able to attend the session as he shared the platform with church leaders from across the world. Just a few days before, I had opened my newspapers to see pictures of the archbishop at the consecration of an unbelieving secular, professor of theology as Bishop of Durham, and three days later, I had seen the pictures after fire had struck causing an estimated million pounds worth of damage to York Minster. However my real purpose was a meeting with the Director of the Christian Medical Commission who took time out from his especially busy schedule. Once again I seemed to be in the right place at the right time. *Document Two*, was available for all who needed it. CMC is a sub-unit of the Programme Unit on Justice and Service, and this report, produced for the distinguished assembly, contained in a nutshell what the Director was able to give me. I learned that in its role as an 'enabler', the CMC purpose is to advise and assist churches and their congregations to combat injustice, to share and to heal, by becoming involved in various 'health promotive approaches.' One of these approaches is the study of Traditional Healing Practices and how they can be integrated with allopathic medicine.

Where then does the CMC stand on alternative (or traditional) medicine? Let the Report★ I was given speak for itself:

'A large part of the world practises and relies on traditional medicines today, and we have much to learn from them. They are based on local culture, and the community plays an important part as the supportive system. There are herbal medicines which are easily available, inexpensive and often very effective alternatives to expensive imported pharmaceuticals. Then there are ancient literature-based systems of medicine, such as acupuncture and acupressure in China, Ayurveda in India, Unani and equally ancient, primal, oral-based indigenous medicine practised in Africa, among the Aborigines of Australia, the Maoris of New Zealand, the Indians of North and South America and the Pacific Islanders.

Over the last decade, the CMC has urged and promoted not only a deeper understanding of traditional healing methods, but also a more effective

★ *Report of Programme Unit (II) on Justice & Service* World Council of Churches, Central Committee, Geneva, Switzerland. 9-18 July 1984

partnership of traditional and allopathic systems of medicine. Traditional medicine has already been recognized and legalized in several countries. Several associations of practitioners of indigenous medicine have been formed around the world; traditional birth attendants (TBAs) are recognized, and training courses building on their skills and utilization are organised both by church agencies and the government.

The study of traditional healing practices and the contribution of traditional healers should continue. Greater attention is also to be given to the spiritual healing and the healing responsibility of the congregation.'

The year 1976 brought in a new era for the WHO. In the same year this neighbour at the WCC also shifted its attention. It moved away from an international perspective to what it calls 'a dynamic search' for the views and understanding of health workers and churches as they confront the situation in their own countries. From 1976 the CMC has sponsored workshops across the world from South East Asia in the east to the Carribean in the west. The results of these have served to bring traditional medicine into focus.

In the WCC bookshop I was offered just two books on healing and the church. One★ described the localised 'search' undertaken by the CMC since 1976. Neither the title of the book nor the apparent purpose of the 'search' seemed to suggest any emphasis on traditional medicine would result, but it is not surprising the discoveries made were in *that* area.

In marked contrast was the other WCC book

★ *The Search for a Christian Understanding of Health, Healing and Wholeness* (Christian Medical Commission, WCC Geneva) - 1982 recommended to me; *The Healing Church,* published twenty years before, was very different in its content. However, whilst very western in its approach, my eyes caught one very small section: 'pre-scientific forms of healing'. That is a small seed that has grown. The search started, and the deception got deeper.

Pre-scientific forms of healing (alternative medicines) are filling the bookshelves today. All that is being written is being consumed by kings and governments, church and state. They seem to have no regard to where the healing comes from.

On a positive note, the WHO has achieved a great deal through medical science and truly natural remedies. No blanket condemnation of the WHO, nor indeed of medical science, is intended in this book, and there is no suggestion that it is wrong for governments and agencies to use the hard-working and caring offices of the WHO. Indeed, its various schemes over the years have, in one area after another, eradicated malaria, yaws and other serious diseases.

PART FOUR
DRUGS AND DOCTORS

18
Why pick on 'alternative medicine'?

This was a question most commonly asked by Christian doctors when I first shared my burden for exposing occult medicine. They have spoken this question from their doubts about medical science, not about 'alternative medicine'. I accept that dependence on drugs in the National Health Service increases, notwithstanding their credibility being in decline. Such is the nature of addiction. My doctor friends are surely right when they say there is much wrong in medicine. I believe there is much that passes for medical science that must be exposed. But I write about 'alternative medicine' because it is a 'growth' business. It is an area that I know!

However, it is sensible briefly to look in on the more familiar medical scene, and I do so in this single chapter.

Drugs first: God second

During my lifetime, we have seen the enormous growth of the pharmaceutical industry and the increased readiness of doctors to prescribe what it offers. It has become normal, even for Christians, to get the medical answer first, and ask God second. Such lack of faith can only put a brake on what He can do.

The pharmaceutical industry is an international one. Research and marketing costs are understandably high. News stories of drugs like Librium and Valium are well-known; commercial considerations are to the fore in a world where Christian values are substantially ignored. Are the pharmaceutical companies perhaps the sorcerers of this age? (Deuteronomy 18: 10-12).

The word 'pharmacy' comes from the Greek *pharmakeia* which means 'enchantment with drugs'. In the Book of Revelation *pharmakios* is always translated 'sorcerer'. Also, what are the origins of medicine itself? The Greek god of medicine is Asklepios (Latin: *Aesculapius)* and the cult of Aesculapius came to Rome in 293 BC when the god (a snake) was established on an island in the Tiber. Rather than the bronze snake God told Moses to set on a pole (Numbers 21:8) this seems the most likely origin of today's medical symbol which includes the serpent!

Drugs are a problem: but beware the wrong answer

In every area of life we can often spot other people's problems in amongst all the confusion; then as laymen we can often bring to them inappropriate answers. The Prince of Wales saw very clearly the problems of the medical profession in Britain during his year as President of the British Medical Association. He said: 'It is frightening how dependent we are all becoming on drugs and how easy it is for doctors to prescribe them as the universal panacea for all ills.'

More than £2,000 million is spent in Britain on drugs in a single year. By and large they only relieve symptoms. They quieten you down, or they prop you up! They bolster your confidence or they quieten your emotions.

Apart from any origins or direct merits of a drug, we have come to know about side-effects. The birth of the thalidomide babies was the foremost example. We were able to *see* the side-effects. Unlike with the thalidomide drug, doctors are in a position to make a value judgement reckoning the side-effects when prescribing steroids. The issues are perhaps difficult for some patients to assess.

However the list of side-effects after the long-term use of steroids is formidable and has given rise to the formation of the 'Steroid Action Aid Group.' They were represented, alongside occult practitioners, at a major exhibition - an alternative medicine exhibition - held in the 'Rainbow Suite' at one of London's major new exhibition centres.

What of the side-effects we don't see? Physical. Emotional. Spiritual. This book is essentially a look at the spiritual dimension; hypnosis opens the way for evil spirits, but what of hypnotic drugs? What actually happens when we are under anaesthetic? Medical science does not try to blind us with an answer. They do not know. The answers to all of these questions are important in spiritual terms.

The British Medical Association (BMA) Report on Alternative Medicine

Back to the alternative medicine scene, taking the doctors' viewpoint the BMA Working Party reported in May 1986. They had been set the task of considering 'the feasibility and possible methods of assessing the value of alternative therapies, whether used alone or to complement other treatments.' Whilst not receiving cooperation from some alternative medicine groups and organisations, the doctors' group set about its task inviting information on the techniques used and on how the various therapies are believed to work. It comprised eight distinguished doctors and had Professor James Payne, Research Professor of Anaesthetics at the Royal College of Surgeons as its chairman.

Copies of 'Understanding Alternative Medicine' (the Second Edition) were received by each member but no questions were asked nor oral evidence invited. However in the report, unlike the World Health Organisation's review of traditional medicine referred to in the previous chapter, there was a page given to 'healing' — supposedly 'divine' healing.

The report on this church-based healing, sandwiched after aromatherapy and Bach flower remedies and before hellerwork, homoeopathy and herbalism, served to throw further light, at any rate for those who have eyes to see, on the Churches Council for Health and Healing already described in Chapter Fifteen of both this book and the previous edition made available to the authors.

The following is an extract from the BMA Report recording the evidence of this body, one seeking to represent different faiths, an extraordinarily difficult task:

"The Working Party also heard oral evidence from the Churches Council for Health and Healing which represents all Christian faiths. They agreed that there had been a revival of consciousness of the healing dimensions of the Ministry. In his evidence Bishop Morris Maddocks said that 20 years ago it would have been difficult for the Churches as a group to have given evidence to the Working Party on 'the renewal of all Churches' consciousness... of the healing dimension of our ministry... This renewal had brought all the Churches together. It has been a healing of the Churches and we have come to a solid mind about these things'. They believed that there should be greater liaison between the church and medicine. Faith was necessary and could complement the treatment given by medical practitioners. Father Joseph di Mauro believed that it was difficult to pinpoint where the faith lay. 'It may be the faith of the practitioner. It may be the faith of the person requesting healing. It may be the faith of the Church, but there has to be faith there.'

In response to a question on the skills of individual healers the Reverend Denis Duncan said that there were certain people with a natural gift that could be used in a particular way. 'It is a gift that not all have... and if one senses, or if a person claims, that they have that gift, I think it is important that there should be some objective authentication of it apart from their own subjective belief.''★

In the light of that statement by the Working Party and of my own report on the Churches Council for Health and Healing set out in Chapter Fifteen, I believe the doctors, not looking from a religious or Christian perspective, could not be faulted for lumping this 'healing' with all the rest of the alternative medicines. The Bible tells us that the things of the Spirit are foolishness to those who do not have the Spirit (1 Corinthians 2: 14). Some medical 'science' may not be science at all, but it must be understood that unredeemed man will expect to find his answers there. The focus of the believer must be on Jesus and we can then discern the source from which the results come. The focus of most doctors is easily set upon results, and if they don't understand the results, they trust and hope that science will provide that answer 'tomorrow'. But even in medical science, let alone in alternative medicine which is our main subject in this book, science may never catch up with phenomena. The

★   *Alternative Therapy - Report of the Board of Science and Education* BMA (1986).

report on alternative medicine disclosed all too little science and its conclusions, but for the odd exception, were a predictable 'thumbs down'. Most of the healing successes of alternative medicine, in the absence of better statistics, are explained away by the one further factor, common in all medicine — the placebo effect.

Hypnosis and hypnotherapy are examples where apart from the Spirit of God the doctors could not be expected to discern the extraordinary dangers, and nor did they. The report tells us:

> 'Although the hypnotic state is not fully understood this should not lead to neglect of hypnosis as a technique as it can benefit certain patients. There is a case for increased research to provide better understanding of hypnotherapy. However, hypnotherapy should only be used as part of the planned management of a condition, and such planned management should always begin with a proper diagnosis. In view of this, the Working Party believes that use of hypnotherapy should be restricted to medical practitioners, dentists and trained and qualified clinical psychologists. ★

It is perhaps the acupuncturists who will have been most satisifed by the report. They can read: 'There is a scientific basis for claims that acupunture is effective as an analgesic.' ★ I must accept that there may well be a scientific basis for the relief of pain by acupuncture. However, before we are as Christians tempted by acupuncture we do well to consider what else might inevitably be involved. Invariably what we have is a mixture. We cannot be reminded too often that Satan is a clever deceiver who will use many ways to catch the unwary. In the words of one journalist specialising in

★ *Alternative Therapy* (BMA - 1986).

medical matters: 'Acupuncture combines the extraordinary with the normal. On the one hand, it is alleged to stimulate a 'vital energy' which is said to run along invisible channels. On the other hand it can to a certain extent be explained in terms of conventional anatomy, and it can be practised by people without extraordinary psychic talents or healing gifts.' ★

It seems from the BMA report that indeed acupuncture can be explained partly in terms of conventional anatomy. But we may well ask where is there to be found a practitioner who has discerned, analysed and dissected the practice and philosophy of acupuncture so as to confine himself only to conventional anatomy? Indeed the result would no longer be acupuncture. To avoid trouble, doctors must start from another place, from whatever science they have established within acupuncture, and not by adopting any of the devil's devices.

So indeed, 'why pick on alternative medicine?' The good and the bad seen in acupuncture by the doctors may be found in drugs too. In this book we are occupied with the subject of alternative medicine. Yet can not drugs also be the wrong kind of medicine?

Drugs: the wrong kind of medicine?

In *The Wrong Kind of Medicine?* ★ ★ it is argued that the power of suggestion is fundamental to all systems of medicine and that medicine works partly just by concentrating the mind on cure. Whilst perhaps most

★ Reproduced from *A Guide to Alternative Medicine* by Robert Eagle (British Broadcasting Corporation, 1980) with the permission of BBC Enterprises Ltd.

★ ★ *The Wrong Kind of Medicine?* by Charles Medawar/Social Audit (Consumer Association - 1984).

drug treatments 'do not benefit patients at all', people underestimate the shortcomings of medicine and are discouraged from thinking about the possible risks and unwarranted effects that are characteristic of virtually all drugs. In this critical guide, Charles Medawar writes that commercial, professional and government interests dominate health care to an extent damaging both to the individual and to national health. The power of suggestion and hope seem to be essential factors to recovery, in the world's view, and Mr Medawar goes some way along the Christian line taken in this book, when he says it is debatable how far drugs should be used to encourage this hope.

As laymen we look for whatever evidence can be found. Two panels of experts, set up to advise an official, public enquiry into the 'Relationship of the Pharmaceutical Industry to the National Health Service' reported as long ago as 1967 that about one third of the most prescribed drug products were officially described as 'undesirable preparations.' That was in a time of soul searching following the birth of the thalidomide babies. What of the not-so-obvious side-effects, and what is the situation today?

The wrong kind of medicine is the natural response to the demands on a doctor to heal. The methods have changed since the days of Adam, but doctors were always successful. This is because whatever is taken in faith can work. Doctors are moving more into alternative therapies, and with the usual faith placed in the doctor these therapies will work especially well when *they* prescribe them.

Doctors understand the power of the placebo referred to previously, and according to the *British Medical Journal* (23 July 1970), analysis of prescriptions in the UK suggests that perhaps one third of all drugs are prescribed for this effect. Placebo is the Latin for 'I will please.' However aren't doctors almost invariably going to prescribe a drug that will have some effect rather than an inert substance coated with sugar? Otherwise, if asked, how could they explain it to the patient? It's well intentioned, but where do these deceptions end? Isn't it urgent that Christians start to put their faith in Jesus and seek to be more alerted to these deceptions as they walk more closely with Him day by day?

It is here that we must part company with Charles Medawar and his most useful book. He has pointed to the most urgent need of an alternative faith; then, towards its end, the book states what an enormous commitment of resources would be needed 'to generate' such an alternative. He points to an alternative faith, not to alternative medicine. I pray he will find it. '...*So then faith cometh by hearing, and hearing by the word of God*' (Romans 10:17).

The doctor's difficult role

If the drug industry has become the sorcerer, has the doctor become something of a 'sorcerer's apprentice'? Doctors are invariably highly intelligent - they have to be to get through their training - and they have been encouraged to focus on the question, 'does it work?' They are not used to approaching 'like a little child' and they are in an extraordinarily difficult situation. On the one hand there are the endless promotions and pressures from the drug companies. On the other they have the demands of an increasing stream of patients; in these days the patients are much less satisfied. Time, patience and solutions are what are really needed, but life has been conditioned by what the drug companies provide. That includes addictive drugs!

Apart from the pharmacology, subject itself to mistakes, when we explore medical science we find that much of it is only theory. A treatment seems to work! It

217

has been tested! So it is repeated! Medicine today is really not as scientific as patients would usually suppose. Consider this up-to-date assessment in a letter written to me by a practising Christian doctor:

While the medical profession today tries to convince itself that there is a very strong scientific basis for all that we do, particularly with the major advances of technology into the field of medicine, I firmly believe this to be a total misnomer. When you begin to explore medicine from a totally scientific viewpoint you find vast, and I mean literally vast, areas of physiology and biochemistry which are not understood at all and much of that which is supposedly understood, is at best theory which as we all know constantly changes. Nowhere is this more than in the area of neuro-physiology and neuro-biochemistry which clearly have direct bearing on the psyche. I feel even in this enlightened twentieth century particularly at general practice level, medicine is as much an art as a science. The good doctor and the brilliant scientist are almost invariably not the same person. In the field of general practice to my mind the best practitioners are those who listen, understand and reassure their patients and can, by affecting the patients attitudes, encourage the inherent healing abilities of the body without recourse to potentially hazardous drugs, whose pharmacology again is often ill understood. Clearly the practitioner must also be aware of that which is illness caused by some pathological process and which indeed can be greatly helped by use of modern drugs and surgical technology, but in my experience this is probably true in less than thirty per cent of cases that a general practitioner will see.

Demons are real; doctors are only human!

How has it happened that believers turn to medicine first and to God second? We have been brought up in a scientific age which has deceived us as to true values. Science has bred materialism with a further distance put between us and God. What science has provided have become gods — motor cars, TVs and all the rest. We have come to depend on them. For our health we have likewise focused on medicine. We have made our doctors into god-figures. We have trusted them. We have respected them. We have believed them. We have thought they knew best. We have believed they were bringing science to us through drugs and their skills. Health has been the most important thing to us - at least when we became ill - and we did as the doctor told us. We have leaned too heavily upon him, and now there is a tendency to blame him! When we have treated the doctor as a god, and indeed when he has responded in such a way, we have only ourselves to blame.

Medicine is changing fast

Medicine is a big and complex subject that falls further into the hands of specialists and experts. At the consultant level we have two dozen or more different specialisations in a big hospital. I have little idea of the drugs or the origins of various treatments. Many of us, like the Prince of Wales, sense that all is not right. The swing to 'alternative medicine' is for every kind of reason. In the 1980 Reith Lecture entitled 'Unmasking Medicine', Ian Kennedy, a legal academic, said: 'The practice of medicine has changed. There's a feeling abroad that all may not be well. This feeling grows out of a sense of distance, out of a sense that medicine is in the hands of the experts and sets its own path. We can take it or leave it.'

Science is relatively new and fifty years ago prior to penicillin, new really effective medical treatments were quite rare. The change we see in Britain has little to do with the founding of the National Health Service after the Second World War. It is a world that laymen find difficulty in entering and understanding. We receive the drug in the simple form of a pill; yet it is so very complicated. Often it defies all understanding. Indeed a drug can be frighteningly spiritual in its effects.

Apart from hypnotic drugs, hypnotism itself is gaining ground and respectability in the medical profession. There is consultation by doctors of psychics for diagnosis; more doctors are discovering the power in psychic 'healing', being led without realising it deeper into the occult realm.

However most doctors can be trusted. The majority are on the side of science and are not into the spiritual! They are only too pleased when the patient ceases to burden them with the god-like image and when he realises his health is substantially in his own hands.

Our health is our reponsibility

Once again the Prince of Wales correctly observed the situation: "The health of human beings is so often determined by their behaviour, their food and the nature of their environment."

We have involved our doctors in everything from conception through to the time when they have to write a certificate to say we are dead! As we hook up to drugs we give up part of our sense of responsibility for our own health. We forget that Satan has a powerful vested interest in our ill-health; the answers suggested by many from the Bible have been far from the truth too.

220

Pointers to the future in the surgery

Of course God can use doctors and we thank Him for all that is achieved through them. Yet the course medicine is assuredly taking today makes our Lord's ways all the more timely for our consideration. 'Why pick on alternative medicine?' was what various doctors asked me when I first embarked on this book. 'What about the state of our own profession?' Yes, indeed!

Many of the drugs are bad enough, but Christians need to be aware that occult alternative therapies appear to be the next step in Satan's plan for the medical profession. Let us take a brief look at the infiltration of blatantly occult alternative therapies into medical science in the United States.

Alternative medicine, whichever way we look at it, has progressed very fast in the past ten years, and the progress is accelerating. It is ten years since it became a recognised subject of teaching in American medical schools. Often teaching will begin with deceptive esoteric technicalities like a description of the human constitution seen in terms of seven states, or levels, of energy. The physical is said to be only the outward manifestation of the lowest form of energy (i.e. matter). The deception runs that in addition to the physical, there are seven more energies that focus on the seven so-called 'chakras' in the body. There is absolutely no scientific basis for the existence of these chakras, and the fact they have been known to occultists for thousands of years doesn't add any credibility to their reality!

The highly regarded John Hopkins Medical School in the United States had opened its door to lecturers in Psychic Healing by 1977★. Whether the classroom is

★ According to *National Enquirer* article: 'Top medical college offers Psychic Healing' (19 July 1977).

there or in any suburban basement room, what we are told when we probe for an explanation, is that we are in another dimension and that all will become clearer when we reach a higher level of consciousness. People with psychic powers turn out to be the ones who provide the evidence. So far so good; for after all, how could the leading 'brains' in a place like John Hopkins, or Oxford, or Cambridge, fall for all this! The truth is, that in these days there are top scientists who are actually *seeking* these psychic powers. Satan, given an opportunity to lumber us with these powers, will do so; now, many are deliberately seeking these powers to apply to their work in research. Such people are believed to have moved into higher levels of evolution. To give them the assurances they may need, demons can, as they are opened up still further, *show* them the energies they had previously learned about. Satan is a legalist, and once we start on the occult trail, he will be aware of his right to encourage us further. We need to walk in the Spirit with our Lord; not with the devil.

America's student doctors today hear how the initiated are able to bypass the normal process of medical science. One such teacher recently had an audience of some 2,000 to 3,000 people, and an estimated sixty per cent of these, according to a report in the *Spiritual Counterfeits Project Journal* of August 1978, were medical professionals. The teacher, a medical doctor, was speaking on the subject of the 'Dynamics of the Etheric-Astral-Mental Fields in the Healing Process'. He saw the future in this way: 'The medical model of the future is one in which a "sensitive" with higher perception is involved with both diagnosis and treatment.' The reality would be diagnosis and treatment in the hands of demons. The warning is worth repeating: we can no longer afford to ignore the spiritual status of those who minister to us whether in the surgery or in the church.

While more and more doctors enthusiastically go

looking for solutions in the spiritual dimension, the vast majority, whether in Britain or in America, busy doing their jobs as well as they can understand them, pay little regard to these alternatives. However, the trend in self-help is not only opening patients to the ideas of alternative medicine; the self-help movement is bringing patients into a different dialogue with doctors. Doctors will learn from their patients! This apart, the doctor is seen much less as a god figure by younger people; the younger doctor has been opened already to the new thinking.

In a book★ published by the World Health Organisation, we are told something about this trend in self-help:

> We are witness to a reorientation in health care provision which might prove as fundamental in the long run as the rise of the medical profession 150 years ago. The key word that symbolises this development is self-help... Self-help encompasses both self-help groups, self-help organisations and alternative care, all of which are part of what as a phenomenon has been referred to as the Self-Help Movement.

The WHO book contains a description of one Patients' Association in England. From the full account given it is clear the relationships between patients and doctors will have benefited. However, and as the WHO Introduction quoted above indicates, self-help incorporates both alternative therapies and these groups. This Patients' Association has had 'about nine evening meetings each year' trying to 'keep a balance between specialist subjects (heart disease, arthritis, acupuncture, marriage

★ *Self-Help and Health in Europe* (WHO - Regional Office for Europe) - 1983.

223

counselling) and more general preventive medicine (eating and health problems of old age, knowing your pills and potions)', and we read that, as a result of the 'talk on yoga' there have been weekly classes for members of the practice for the past three years.

We know that if we keep our eyes open we see there are talks on yoga followed by yoga classes held in many different places. However the concern here must be with the overtures Satan is making, not only in encouraging the out-and-out searchers amongst the doctors, but also to the hardheaded, hard working general practitioner who has neither the time nor inclination to go to lectures on subjects like 'Dynamics of the Etheric-Astral-Mental Fields in the Healing Process'.

There are more ways than one of getting yoga, acupuncture and all the rest closer, and then *into,* the surgery of every doctor. Patients' associations and self-help groups seem to be one more way. The idea of these groups is good. As ever, Satan much prefers to work through something that is good.

Satan has his answers all ready

Satan - the planner - is ready. He says, "You have looked outside of yourself for the answer, and you haven't found it in science and drugs". So now he says, "Look to yourself for the answer. It's very simple. The answer was there all the time. The ancient peoples understood it. But you've been too busy with science". "Look at the natural things" he would say to us. "Look to homoeopathy with its herbs and its minerals! Go to work on those energy lines in your body that even the ancient Chinese could understand! Look at the psychic powers you can develop!" What Satan doesn't whisper is that drugs have helped prepare our spirits for the 'alternative medicine' scene. We have been conditioned for a reaction to the wonder drugs. Now the emphasis is shifting to so-called natural mixtures and potions; going deeper than just the symptoms; practitioners with more time to spare; the 'whole person' treatment; diet, exercise and personal responsibility; no side-effects - a carefully prepared mixture of the counterfeit and the beneficial with just about the right dosage in line with what the patient will take.

A born again rector of a busy parish put it this way in a letter to me:

> The pressures on doctors to cope with demands on them mean they can only give each patient an average six minutes each! Hence people's dissatisfaction with orthodox medicine has turned them to those who will give them what they really want (they think!) which is more time for someone to treat them as a person not a number. So often the people filling this gap are precisely those outlined (referring to the sort of therapies seen in Part Two). Hence the need for Christians to lead people to find that sense of whole-ness and self-value which is only ours through the love of God the Father revealed in the Son Jesus Christ and lived in the power of the Holy Spirit. Physical healing is only a very small part of what we need.

Healing can be found in Jesus. Against that, man is being wooed by the powers of darkness in 'alternative medicine'. There is spiritual warfare, and Satan's 'simple' answer is the counterfeit of the most simple answer of all — to receive the wholeness and life that Jesus is able to give us.

19
Moral Rearmament health conference

I sent out one hundred letters and trusted I would be covered by prayer as I attended a Health Care Conference promoted by Moral Rearmament, in Switzerland. The time was spiritually debilitating much as I anticipated, but it had seemed to be right that I go.

I had been to one previous World Assembly of MRA, but this would be my only visit as a born again believer. Would I really find any born again people there? Would I find any believers to whom I could relate in the medical field? How would I find MRA now that I knew Jesus, now I knew that He was the Healer?

I found *many* born again believers. Furthermore many of them were seeking so evidently actually to *live* moral lives, the sort of lives they had found generally lacking in many of the traditional churches they had known. However there were many at the conference who will never have heard the gospel of Jesus.

Since its foundation, I believe the movement was taken out of balance by its focus on the absolute moral standards of love, honesty, unselfishness and purity, rather than on the person of Jesus. Certainly I found no focus on Jesus in 1984.

Unlike my visit three years earlier, being now a Christian, I was sensitive to much that was led by the spirit of Antichrist and the New Age. One lovely man whom I knew from previous meetings, to reinforce a point he was making to me, said 'We should ask the tree before we cut it down.'

The Dalai Lama was quoted approvingly by the British general practitioner who opened the conference. The Tibetan Buddhist leader was at that time touring Britain and being widely received by church leaders as a spokesman for ecumenism and religious tolerance. More significantly in the New Age, there can be seen in the Dalai Lama a missionary zeal that is both subtle and unexpected from the eastern religions. This **Buddhist** spiritual leader was the president of the 1979 World **Hindu** Conference. Ecumenism and compromise are not only gaining ground in the west, but in the east too.

At the same introductory session we were encouraged by a Moslem, 'Don't fall into the trap of seeing only one God.' Everything but the Bible seemed to be quoted. 'We all have this priceless gift of inner intelligence,' the speaker said. Another platform speaker said, 'I was scientific, then I discovered the writings of old doctors.' 'The great doctor, Paracelsus,' didn't of course escape the conference's mention. I heard another say, 'We are one family at this conference, breathing through one another,' but this was not a Christian conference where there is a unity that comes from the focus of all on Jesus.

This movement seemed to have deteriorated by a long stretch since Frank Buchman founded it as the Oxford Group following upon his conversion at the Keswick Convention more than fifty years previously. As ever Satan built upon what was good. Still he works on that principle today. 'In my religion abortion is strictly forbidden,' one of the principal speakers told us. 'This gives me a completely new view and respect for Islam,' was the reply of one well respected speaker, and when the distinguished Muslim was seated, a medical doctor from Canada, whom I knew, led the large assembly in a standing ovation. This man was a principal speaker too. He was the former doctor of Frank Buchman. He was also the joint author of *Remaking Men,* my 'bible' when I was a New Ager.

I had fellowshipped mostly with the Hindus, who were much in evidence, at the previous conference. Perhaps it was a sign of the times that the principal contributor at this conference (made up of entirely orthodox medical personnel rather than those from the alternative therapies) was an Egyptian from oil-rich Kuwait. The doctor hadn't given us anything from the Bible, but the medical professor from the University of Kuwait, and whose idea the conference was, gave us quotations from the Koran. Here was a really attractive man with peace, morality and kindness shining out from him, and it was his job to address us on 'Moral and Ethical Issues.' But he didn't know that Jesus Christ was the only way to the Father.

As I observe the resolute way in which believers and others, whether in their own strengths or in any other way, live by these attractive moral standards, and how they influence the lives of others, I see how subtle it is, and how easy it can be to stray when we take our eyes off Jesus. My thoughts turned to the wider New Age scene as the religions and cults like MRA prepare the ground for the peace, unity and supernatural power that the world is seeking. It is not the unity of believers, nor that peace that passes all understanding. It is the peace that the world and the cults can give, and the power promises to be the power of the occult.

All of the speakers were orthodox medical men and women, and it was a Swiss psychiatrist, who stirred the most approval with what seemed to be a confused mixture of psychiatry, theology and the occult. The contents were the ingredients so readily recognised by those who are at all familiar with Satan's ways in these days: '... he should practise the maximum possible physical and mental inactivity... composure, Maryan openness, and self-critical humility towards the workings of God's

229

grace.' Jesus came to give life and we are not to be left wide open to demon activity by this sort of meditative contemplation. Jesus came so that we can have a real relationship with Him, and not listen to the repetitive and rhythmic prayers the professor described as part of his treatments.

Another therapy this psychiatrist had developed was what he called, 'a three year course of prayer in basic psychosomatic therapy.' He concluded: 'I have often found that people who have finished their final period of three years' therapy do not want to give up the searching, transforming, praying and thanking way to God.' His observation is correct! But we search at our peril! They *may* find their way to God. The only way is through Jesus. No search is necessary. Jesus is just a prayer away!

The MRA Health Care Conference made a small yet significant contribution to New Age health care. Orthodox medical practitioners were discovering there *is* a spiritual way. Yet the only spiritual way they dare take is the way that is with Jesus, *'for there shall arise false Christs, and false prophets, and shall shew great signs and wonders; insomuch that, if it were possible, they shall deceive the very elect. Behold I have told you before'* (Matthew 24:24-25).

20
The Bible's medical answers

The Bible has given doctors the answers in the past

Let us see the contribution the Bible makes into the area of preventive medicine. S I McMillen MD, in *None of these Diseases*★ relates how the Black Death was brought under control. He tells us that in the fourteenth century alone this killer disease took the lives of one in four people, an estimated total of sixty million. Then the church set about separating the afflicted according to God's word in Leviticus 13: 46: *'All the days wherein the plague shall be in him he shall be defiled; he is unclean: he shall dwell alone; without the camp shall his habitation be'*

We can take a look back at the nineteenth century when there were epidemics of cholera and typhoid through the dumping of human excrement in the streets. God promised Moses that the Israelites in Egypt would have none of these diseases (Exodus 15: 26). However there was something *they* had to do and it was written in Deuteronomy 23:12-13: *'Thou shalt have a place also without the camp, whither thou shalt go forth abroad.'* Could the Lord have made it any plainer? However He was ignored by the grand designers in places like Florence and Vienna where there was little concern for the open sewers.

★ Published by Marshall, Morgan & Scott - 1966

The Bible today

The Bible is a supernatural book, always providing the answer; practical and up-to-date. More and more are devoted to the counterfeit answers provided by horoscopes, but for increasing numbers with eyes to see and ears to hear, the Bible gives the only truth that can be found. Today alcohol is a major killer and the word of God contains the truth about it. Proverbs 23: 31-32 says: *'Look not thou upon the wine when it is red, when it giveth his colour in the cup, when it moveth itself aright. At the last it biteth like a serpent, and stingeth like an adder.'*

Lung cancer and coronary heart disease, both brought on by smoking, are major killers. We have all seen medical pictures of lungs destroyed by inhaled smoke. In 1 Corinthians 6: 19 we can read: *'What? know ye not that your body is the temple of the Holy Ghost which is in you, which ye have of God, and ye are not your own?'*

Venereal disease, little discussed in 'polite society', is nonetheless a prevalent and most dreadful disease. Proverbs 5: 3-5 has this to say: *'For the lips of a strange woman drop as an honeycomb, and her mouth is smoother than oil: But her end is bitter as wormwood, sharp as a two-edged sword. Her feet go down to death; her steps take hold on hell.'*

And what of our minds, diseased through following our own inclinations and not allowing the Holy Spirit to provide the essential love, joy and peace? Paul told the Galatians what any good doctor would suggest we avoid to promote good physical and mental health. Galatians 5: 19-21 says: *'Now the works of the flesh are manifest, which are these; Adultery, fornication, uncleanness, lasciviousness, idolatry, witchcraft, hatred, variance, emulations, wrath, strife, seditions, heresies, envyings, murders, drunkenness, revellings, and such like:'* Satan is the author of disorders that are brought about through these sinful acts, and these disorders where no pathology or tissue disease is evidenced, amount, according to general practitioners, for some seventy per cent or so of the patients coming to them.

The Bible has much to say about Satan, the source of occult power and the author of disease. It is because of our sinful nature that we are subject to sickness. We have seen that Satan is the power behind many alternative healing methods. Often he is the power behind accidents and much else besides. He is the enemy encouraging the sinful nature that gives rise to the majority of bodily afflictions. How then can Christians deal with Satan when he makes a personal attack?

We need to know Satan

In one sense I knew Satan and his power through my 'search' into alternative medicine, and before I knew Jesus as my Saviour and Lord. I believe many spend twenty years or so going to church - as I did - before really **knowing** Jesus. Then, for need of teaching and because Satan blinds, they can easily spend another twenty years and still not **know** Satan. The enemy is not 'evil'. The enemy is a personality - Satan.

Isn't it better not to think about the enemy? Satan himself plants that question in many minds. When our soldiers were doing battle against Germany in Europe, they weren't concentrating on the evil of Nazi philosophy and of Hitler, but on the enemy that confronted them. Like them, Christians have a battle on their hands and we have to **know** the enemy. The Bible tells us in Ephesians 6: 12 that our battle is not against flesh and blood but against Satan's spiritual forces. In the battle against Hitler, our leaders had to understand his tactics as best as they could, and our military officers took account of them on the battle field. In the battle against Satan we can know his tactics because the Bible reveals them to us.

The Bible says that Satan attacks viciously (1 Peter 5:8). He takes advantage of human weakness (2 Cor. 2:11), and he blinds our spiritual vision (2 Cor. 4:4). He seeks to bind us physically, mentally and spiritually (Luke 13:16; Acts 10:38). Satan is a counterfeiter (Acts 8:9-11), who deceives all men (Rev. 12:9; 2 Cor. 11:14ff). He hinders the gospel (2 Thess. 2:7-10); he steals the truth (Matt. 13:19; John 10:10); he afflicts and destroys (Job 2:3-6; John 10:10); he is a liar and can't be trusted (Acts 5:3; 1 John 2:22). Satan's demons can indwell both humans and animals (Matt. 8:31ff). Satan accuses humanity, and Christians in particular (Zech. 3). He tempts all to sin (Luke 22:31; Matt 16:22ff), and he is interested in governments too (Dan. 10:10-13; 12:1; Rev. 13).

Jesus has already won the victory on the cross, and He is with us in our battles. However *we* do the fighting. We need to get light focused on the enemy, heed what God says about him and not be afraid to talk to others about him. We need to have a healthy respect for him. We are much safer when we know him as Jesus knew him, and in the light of what God says about him.

We need to watch out for Satan

He seeks to inspire in us the wickedness so well

summarised in the letter of Paul to the Galatians already referred to in this chapter. Accordingly we have to watch out for him. *'Watch and pray, that ye enter not into temptation: the spirit indeed is willing, but the flesh is weak'* (Matthew 26:41).

Satan is at work in the area of our health. We have seen that he is at work in the area of alternative medicine. There is not one of his tactics referred to above that he could not use in these areas, but we can be ready for him when he first puts that sinful thought into our minds or when we first start to doubt God's word.

The attack might be a worry or a fear, a thought of dissatisfaction, gossip or laziness, a jealous idea, a feeling of pride, or, in the context of health, a doubt that our Lord is the Lord who is able to heal. The list, encouraged by Satan and forbidden by God, is a long one, but the Holy Spirit always dwells within us. We can allow ourselves to be led by Him.

OTHER BOOKS BY ROY LIVESEY

Trade Orders:
New Wine Press,
PO Box 17,
Chichester PO20 6YB
England

Overseas:
c/o 3 College St, Wendouree, Vic 3355 Australia
c/o PO Box 24086, Royal Oak, Auckland, New Zealand
c/o 14 Balmoral Road, Singapore 1025
c/o PO Box 1613, Cape Town 8000, South Africa

ROY AND RAE LIVESEY

are distributors of

'THE PRINCE AND THE PARANORMAL'
by John Dale

(1987 – 256 pages, £3.50)

This is an important book which follows the 'search' of Prince Charles in the New Age.

It presents an excellent insight into the New Age through a review of the long Royal involvement in the Paranormal, and it evidences the need to pray for our rulers.

Personal orders for this book, for the books on the following pages, and details of **THE NEW AGE BULLETIN** will be supplied to those who write to:

Roy & Rae Livesey,
Bury House,
Clows Top,
Kidderminster,
Worcs DY14 9HX,
England.

Please add 10% for U.K. postage.

NEW AGE TO NEW BIRTH

A Personal Testimony of Two Kingdoms
(Roy and Rae Livesey)

- Experiences in the New Age Movement and the Occult realm
- Exposing Satan's wiles as a Christian
- Looking at Meditation, Divination, Moral Re-Armament, Rock Music, Healing and Ley-Lines

ROY LIVESEY sought a better world and more worthwhile life through Politics, Church-going, Meditation, Peace, Ecology and Moral Re-Armament. Eventually the ways of the NEW AGE led him to counterfeit healing in Satan's supernatural realm. Despite his good intentions he didn't know that Satan could masquerade as an angel of light. *(2 Corinthians 11:14).*

This is a personal story of TWO KINGDOMS. In one Roy found Satan's deceptions throught Leylines, Divination, Occult Healing and Moral Re-Armament. Then he received the NEW BIRTH and with it the discernment of these deceptions. Indeed he found them not only in the New Age movement but in the Body of Christ itself.

Except for a single chapter written by Rae, it is substantially written from Roy's personal experiences. Yet Roy and Rae were in the story together. *(Matthew 19:4-5).*

192 pages   £2.50
New Wine Press, 1986   ISBN 0 947852 16 6

UNDERSTANDING THE NEW AGE

World Government and World Religion

- a Different book on Rome and the Jesuits
- a Different look at the Bankers, Credit and the 'Love of Money'
- a Different perspective on Conspiracy

Few writers about the New Age have described the secret internationalist groups, built up through the love of money (1 Timothy 6:10). Then amid the deception of the New Age Babylon few today recognise the hand of MYSTERY BABYLON THE GREAT, THE MOTHER OF HARLOTS described in Revelation 17.

This Second Edition explores these vital areas and deals with groups building the New World Order. The separate volume, 'More Understanding the New Age', deals with the New Age deception of the individual.

This book gives an insight into the pieces of the jigsaw, which while apparently unconnected do fit together to give a picture of the planned New Age.

It is a warning to the Church to be watchmen and discern the times and seasons in which we live, redeeming the time for the days are evil.

Roy Livesey is uniquely qualified to comment on this difficult subject, having been involved in many New Age organisations before his conversion and writes with much first hand experience.

218 pages   £3.50
New Wine Press, 1989   ISBN 0 947852 26 3

MORE UNDERSTANDING THE NEW AGE

Discerning Antichrist and the Occult Revival

- Identifying ways individuals are deceived in the New Age
- The move towards One-World Faith
- A call for Christians to use more discernment

History of the New Age. New Age Centres and Leaders. The Occult in the New Age. New Age One-world faith. Christians and the New Age.

This is a companion volume to 'Understanding the New Age – World Government and World Religion', which deals with the building of the New World Order.

160 pages   £2.95
New Wine Press, 1990   ISBN 0 947852 62 X

UNDERSTANDING DECEPTION

New Age Teaching in the Church

- Highlighting the Deception in the Church
- A Plea to Check the Current Winds of Doctrine
- Warning Christians who would Build a Kingdom on Earth

We are warned that in the last days the Church will be faced with doctrines which are demonically inspired and which seek to deceive even God's chosen people. While appearing to be Biblical at first glance many have their roots either in secular psychology, self-improvement teaching, Eastern religions or the occult. Despite being incompatible with what Jesus taught they are nevertheless promoted in a Christianised form as new revelations by well respected Bible teachers.

This book is a plea to check the current winds of doctrine with what Jesus Himself taught and to discern those errors incorporated in the new doctrines that abound.

Roy Livesey writes from personal experience and involvement in New Age groups.

224 pages   £3.50
New Wine Press, 1990   ISBN 0 947852 29 8

INDEX

**Note: Further names are to be found in the checklist
of cults and the occult on pages 129-134.**

B

Hunt, Dave   85, 138, 191, 192, 193, 194
hydrotherapy   67
hypnosis   28, 75, 83, 86, 116, 164, 174, 211, 214, 220
hypnotherapy   67, 75, 214

I

Imam Mahdi   156
imagination   86, 191
India   52, 54, 96, 140, 147, 164
Indian boxing   54
inherited powers   99
inner healing   15, 87, 186, 188, 189, 194
interpersonal relationship   90
ionisation therapy   65
iridology   100, 105

J

Japan   54, 55, 67
Jehovahs Witnesses   155
Jin Shin Do   50
Journal of Alternative Medicine   195, 196
John Hopkins Medical School   221
Judge, WQ   147
judo   54
Jung   87, 174, 191

K

karate   54
Kendall, Dr RT   109
Kennedy, Ian   219
Kentian Homoeopathy   121
Kent, James Tyler   122
kinesiology   96, 97, 105
Kirlian photography   100, 105, 158

O

P